THE ESSENTIAL FOODS LISTS FOR THE GLYCEMIC INDEX DIET

DISCOVER THE FOODS SCIENTIFICALLY PROVEN TO PROMOTE WEIGHT LOSS AND OVERALL HEALTH — WITH THE GI VALUES OF OVER 2000 FOODS

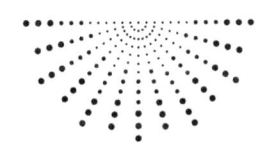

DR. H. MAHER

Copyright © 2020 "The Essential Foods Lists for the Glycemic Index Diet" by Dr. H. Maher

All rights reserved.

ISBN: 9798445139867

Under no circumstances will any legal responsibility or blame be held against the publisher for any reparation, damages, or monetary loss due to the information herein, either directly or indirectly.

Legal Notice:

All rights reserved. No portion of this book may be reproduced, stored in a retrieval system, or transmitted in any form or by any means—electronic, mechanical, photocopy, recording, scanning, or other—except for brief quotations in critical reviews or articles, without the prior written permission of the publisher.

Medical Disclaimer: Because each individual is different and has particular dietary needs or restrictions, the dieting and nutritional information provided in this book does not constitute professional advice and is not a substitute for expert medical advice. Individuals should always check with a doctor before undertaking "a dieting, weight loss, or exercise regimen and should continue only under a doctor's supervision. While we provide the advice and information in this book in the hopes of helping individuals improve their overall health, multiple factors influence a person's results, and individual results may vary. When a doctor's advice to a particular individual conflicts with advice provided in this book, that individual should always follow the doctor's advice. Patients should not stop taking any of their medications without the consultation of their physician.

❦ Created with Vellum

CONTENTS

Introduction										v

Part I
THE GLYCEMIC INDEX DIET : OVERVIEW & GUIDELINES
1. The Low-Glycemic Diet for Weight Loss						3
2. Carbohydrates, Proteins and Fats: How do macronutrients fit into a healthy low-glycemic diet?	19
3. Food, weight loss and Diabetes							32
4. Foods to Include in your Low Glycemic Diet					38
5. Eating Low Glycemic and Anti-Inflammatory Foods				44
6. Avoiding High Glycemic and Inflammatory Foods				50
7. Eating Whole and minimally Processed foods					54
8. 12 Principles & Tips of Low-glycemic Eating					57
9. Meal Planning Guidelines							70

Part II
YOUR GROCERY SHOPPING LIST FOR LOW GI FOODS
10. Portions & Serving Sizes							89
11. Beverages: Low and Medium Glycemic Index Foods				104
12. Breads: Low and Medium Glycemic Index Foods				114
13. Dairy and alternatives: Low and Medium Glycemic Index Foods		131
14. Fish and Seafood: Low and Medium Glycemic Index Foods			145
15. Fruits: Low and Medium Glycemic Index Foods				150
16. Grains: Low and Medium Glycemic Index Foods				156
17. Legumes: Low and Medium Glycemic Index Foods				161
18. Meats and Poultry: Low and Medium Glycemic Index Foods			165
19. Mixed Meals and Convenience Foods						189
20. Soups: Low and Medium Glycemic Index Foods				202

21. Sauces, Oils and Salad Dressing: Low and Medium 211
    Glycemic Index Foods
22. Spices and Herbs: Low and Medium Glycemic Index Foods 217
23. Vegetables: Low and Medium Glycemic Index Foods 220

Health and Nutrition Websites 235
About the Author 237

INTRODUCTION

The Glycemic Index Diet is a powerful tool to help you understand the impact of carbohydrates on your blood sugar levels and can help you achieve sustainable weight loss and improved health. By focusing on low-glycemic foods, you can maintain your blood sugar levels stable, reduce cravings and hunger, and achieve a healthier, more balanced diet.

The Low-Glycemic Diet is a powerful diet with proven results for weight loss, weight management, diabetes control, diabetes prevention, and heart disease. It provides a diet plan and general nutritional guidelines on how foods affect your blood sugar levels.

The Glycemic Index (GI) was originally developed in the early 1980s to scientifically determine how different carbohydrate-containing foods—vegetables, legumes, fruits, processed foods, and dairy products— affect blood sugar levels. Since Dr. Jenkins' initial research more than 35 years ago, many scientists have recognized the potential

INTRODUCTION

of the GI as a powerful tool for managing weight, improving the effectiveness of weight loss diets, and managing diabetes.

The GI isn't formally a diet in the sense that you have to follow strict rules and specific meal plans or eliminate certain foods from your daily diet. Instead, it's a scientific way of identifying how carbohydrates affect blood sugar levels and measuring how slowly or quickly the carbohydrates in foods raise blood sugar. As a result, the glycemic index is fundamental to knowing whether you want to maintain weight, lose weight, and better control diabetes and certain health problems.

The "Glycemic Index (GI) Diet" refers to a targeted eating plan that uses the Glycemic Index as the primary and only guiding principle for meal planning. Unlike other diet plans that provide a strict recommendation with specific proportions, the GI Diet does not specify the optimal daily number of calories, amount of carbohydrates, protein, or fat for weight maintenance or weight loss, but provides an effective eating plan with more flexibility and sustainable results for weight loss, weight management, and diabetes control.

WHAT IS THE GLYCEMIC INDEX?

Dr. Jenkins first created the Glycemic Index in the early 1980s to help people with diabetes effectively control and manage their blood glucose levels. The original work involved analyzing 60 foods and measuring how slowly or quickly the foods caused blood sugar levels to rise. The glycemic index is essential to health because high blood sugar spikes can lead to kidney failure or cardiovascular disease. Foods with a low glycemic index release glucose into the blood slowly and evenly. Conversely, foods with a high glycemic index release glucose quickly.

Since this initial work, researchers have found that foods with a low glycemic index (low GI foods) are ideal for weight loss diets and promote weight loss, in addition to their beneficial effects on the pancreas (insulin release), eyes, and kidneys.

The GI is calculated on a scale of 1 to 100. Each food is assigned a score on this scale based on experimental data. A lower score indicates that the food takes a long time to raise blood sugar levels.

Complex carbohydrates are superior to starchy and refined carbohydrates in weight loss and weight gain prevention diets. An excellent way to differentiate healthy carbohydrates is by their glycemic index.

UNDERSTANDING GI VALUES

Glycemic index (GI) values are divided into three categories:

- Low GI: This category includes foods with a GI of less than 55.
- Medium GI: This category includes foods with a GI between 56 and 69.
- High GI: In general, this category should be avoided because the foods cause high spikes in blood sugar levels. They have a GI of 70 or higher.

Comparing GI values can help guide your food choices. For example, muesli has a GI of about 86. A fruit and vegetable smoothie has on a GI of 55.

HOW IS THE GLYCEMIC INDEX MEASURED?

The GI values of foods are measured using valid and proven scientific methods and cannot be guessed by looking at the composition of a particular food or the nutritional information on food packaging.

Therefore, the GI calculation follows the international standard method and provides values that are generally accepted. The GI of a food is calculated by feeding more than ten healthy people a portion of the test food containing fifty grams of digestible carbohydrate and then measuring the effect on each participant's blood glucose levels (blood glucose response) over the next two hours.

In the second part of the process, the same participants are given the same carbohydrate portion of glucose (used as a reference food) and their blood glucose response is measured over the next two hours.

The GI value for the food is then calculated for each participant using a simple formula (dividing the blood glucose response to the food by the blood glucose response to the glucose (reference food)). The final GI value for the food is the average GI value for the participants (over 10).

Carbohydrates with a low GI (55 or less) are digested, absorbed, and metabolized more slowly and cause a smaller and slower rise in blood glucose and, therefore, usually insulin levels.

Low glycemic diets or foods are associated with a reduced risk of chronic disease. Foods with low glycemic indexes are known for their ability to release glucose into the blood slowly and evenly. Conversely, foods with a high glycemic index are known to release glucose rapidly. Research suggests that foods with a low glycemic index (LGI foods) are ideal for weight loss diets and promote sustained weight loss, in addition to their beneficial effects on the pancreas (insulin release), eyes, and kidneys.

THE GLYCEMIC LOAD CONCEPT

Basing food choices solely on GI means focusing on one aspect, the quality of the carbohydrates in the food, and ignoring another equally important aspect, the quantity of carbohydrates in the food. Hence the importance of glycemic load, which combines these two criteria and, when available, provides a more sophisticated tool for better weight loss control and effective diabetes management.

INTRODUCTION

The glycemic load was later developed by Harvard researchers to provide a more useful tool for tracking both the quality of carbohydrates. The glycemic load of a given food has direct physiological significance in that each unit of GL is equivalent to the glycemic effect of consuming 1 g of glucose. Typical low glycemic diets contain 80-150 GL units per day. **If you have diabetes, you can consume up to 50 grams of sugar per day (from all sources) based on a 2,000-calorie diet. This means you should aim for a GL of 50.**

The glycemic load (GL) is calculated using the following formula:

Glycemic Load (GL) = GI x Net Carbohydrates (grams) content per portion ÷ 100

Where net carbohydrate = total carbohydrates - dietary fiber

GLYCEMIC LOAD RANGES

Like the glycemic index, the glycemic load (GL) of a food can be classified as

- Low: 10 or less
- Medium: 11 - 19
- High: 20 or more

For a standard serving size of food, the glycemic load (GL) is considered high if the GL is greater than or equal to 20, moderate if the GL is in the range of 11-19, and low if the GL is less than or equal to 10. Daily GL is the sum of the GLs for all foods consumed during the day.

INTRODUCTION

SHOULD I USE THE GI OR THE GL?

You don't need to calculate or track the glycemic index (GL) of your meals. Although the concept of glycemic load (GL) is useful and well-documented in scientific research, and integrates both the quality and quantity of the carbs you eat. You can use interchangeably the glycemic index (GI) or glycemic load, provided that if you follow the glycemic index diet, you must stick to the portions and serving sizes to keep the amounts of carbohydrates you eat in line with your personal needs.

The use of the GI seems more intuitive and simple than the GL, in the sense that if you use the GI as it was originally intended—to select the lowest GI food within a meal group or food category—you will most likely select the food with the lowest glycemic index, assuming you eat a standard portion size. Foods are grouped together based on similar nutrients (carbohydrate, protein, fat, vitamins) and similar amounts of carbohydrate. **If you then choose healthy foods according to their low GI values, <u>at least 70% at each meal</u>, chances are you are following an eating plan that not only keeps your blood glucose at the safest level, but also contains balanced amounts of essential nutrients—carbohydrates, proteins and fats.**

WILL GLYCEMIC INDEX (GI) DIET HELP YOU LOSE WEIGHT?

Glycemic index diets show much more weight loss in the short and medium term than other diets. Eating foods with a low glycemic index (GI) is the key to weight loss and hormone balance. A 2012 study published in the Journal of the American Medical Association found that low glycemic index (low GI) diets were best and superior at maintaining weight loss when compared to very low carbohydrate diets (such as the ketogenic or keto diet) and low-fat diets. The findings support the GI diet's assertion that "a calorie is not a calorie" and that "different types of foods affect us in different ways, despite having the same number of calories". Another study published in 2014 in The American Journal of Clinical Nutrition supports low glycemic and calorie-restricted diets as more effective than high glycemic and low-fat diets for weight management and weight loss.

PART I
THE GLYCEMIC INDEX DIET : OVERVIEW & GUIDELINES

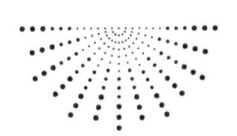

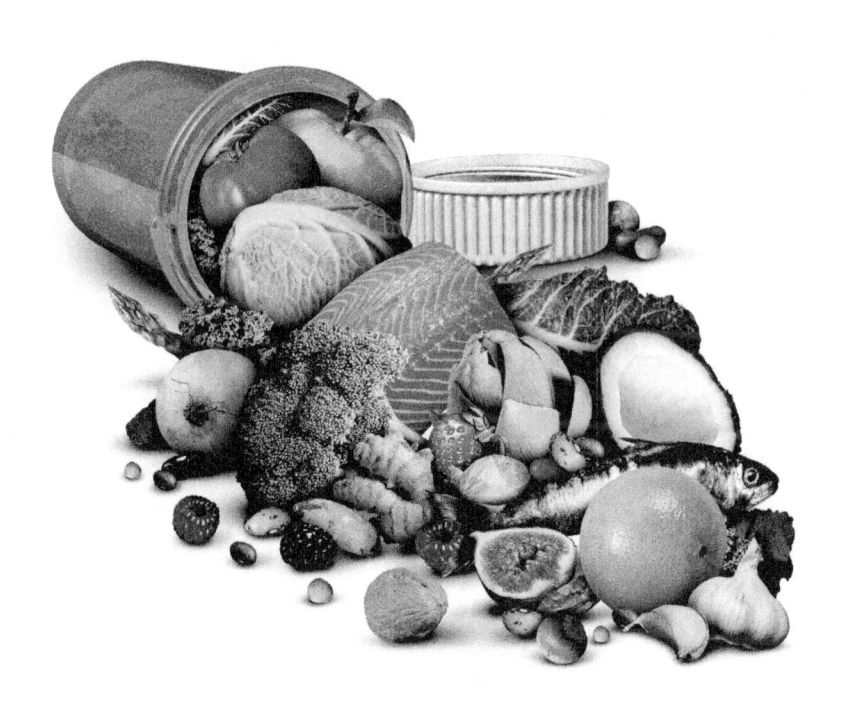

1
THE LOW-GLYCEMIC DIET FOR WEIGHT LOSS

If you search for low-GI diets online, you'll find a lot of promising weight-loss miracles along without any evidence-based science or related research. Suppose you decide to go further and try to implement such methods. In that case, you will be sure to run into flaws and inconsistencies because the GI diet, unlike many other diets, didn't provide formal guidelines nor provide optimal daily foods intake as many claims.

Keeping in mind that the glycemic index diet is instead an eating plan or a lifestyle will increase your awareness of achieving a lasting weight loss or maintaining a healthy condition by eating according to the glycemic index.

Fortunately, the science behind weight loss is today better developed, especially the link between hormones and weight gain and obesity. Therefore, if you intend to achieve a healthy weight, you have to understand how some specific hormones are involved in the weight gain process and how to make them work for you by eating good carbohydrates (low-GI foods).

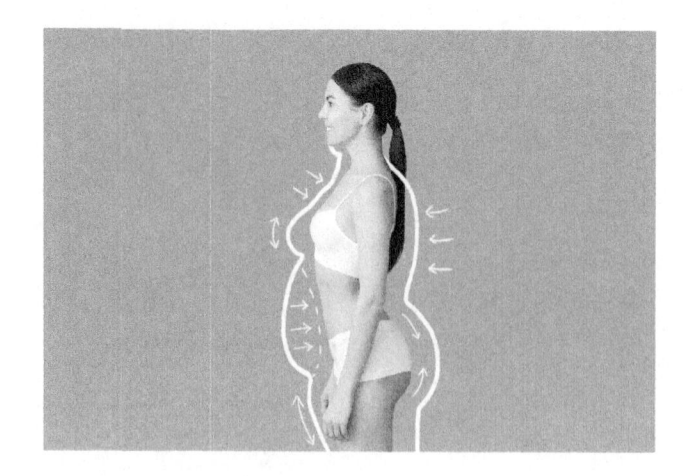

This first part of this chapter will discuss the legitimate science behind weight gain, satiety, anger, hormones and show you how incorporating low-GI foods into your daily intakes is the masterpiece of the weight-loss process. Because those high-quality foods will help minimize cravings, reduce the risk of insulin resistance, and suppress your appetite.

HORMONES THAT REGULATE BODY WEIGHT

1- THE INSULIN HORMONE

Insulin is the most important hormone produced by the pancreas. It regulates glucose absorption by body cells and maintains the level of blood sugar in a healthy range. When you ingest foods, they travel to your stomach and intestines to be broken down into micronutrients. The pancreas releases insulin to enable body cells to absorb and transform sugar into energy throughout the body.

Insulin also signals to the liver, muscle, and adipocytes (fat cells) to store the excess glucose for further use. Extra sugar is stored in 3 ways:

- In muscle tissues in the form of glycogen.
- In the liver in the form of glycogen.
- In adipose tissue (fat reserves of the body) in the form of triglycerides which are fat molecules that store energy

WEIGHT GAIN AND INSULIN

In theory, it's impossible to gain weight if you eat no carbohydrates because the pancreas will not release insulin, the only polypeptide hormone that induces fat storage into adipose tissue. And thus, you can not have any more fat stored in your body. So, if you want to lose weight, it's essential that rises and falls in blood sugar must be as smooth as possible. The longer the digestion of carbohydrates takes, the better it is. And here came the importance of the glycemic index concept.

Remember that eating high glycemic index food cause a rapid rise in insulin hormone levels in the blood, translating to excess fat in the body. Insulin is the hormone that sends sugar out of the bloodstream into the tissue cells for use as energy. When extra sugar resides in the blood, insulin hormone levels stay high, and insulin sends the signal to the body to store excess calories in the form of fat. Thus, High insulin hormone levels imply you'll have more body fat, while low insulin hormone levels mean you'll have less body fat.

INSULIN RESISTANCE

Insulin resistance is a serious and silent health condition that occurs when cells in your muscles, liver, and body fat start ignoring the signal that insulin is sending out to transfer glucose out of the blood. As insulin resistance develops, the body reacts by producing more and more insulin to lower blood sugar.

Over time, the β cells in the pancreas working hard to make a higher supply of insulin can no longer provide more and more insulin. Your blood sugar may reflect the pancreas failure to maintain the level in the healthy range, and your blood sugar rises, showing pre-diabetes or, at worst, diabetes type 2.

Insulin resistance is silent and presents no symptoms in the first stage of its development. The symptoms appear later when the condition worsens, and the pancreas cannot produce enough insulin to maintain your blood sugar within the healthy range. When this occurs, the symptoms may be severe including, metabolic syndrome, polycystic ovary syndrome (PCOS), and various types of diabetes.

Fortunately, it is possible to reduce the effects of insulin resistance and boost your insulin sensitivity by following a low-glycemic index diet.

Thus, for many of you, following a low-glycemic diet goes beyond weight-loss management and target the management of particular health condition sensitive to such kind of diet and particularly those related to insulin resistance like:

- Excessive hunger
- Lethargy or tiredness
- Difficulty concentrating
- Brain fog
- Waist weight gain
- High blood pressure

Can insulin resistance be reduced or reversed?

Fortunately, It is possible to reduce the effects of insulin resistance and boost your insulin sensitivity by following some effective methods, including:

- Low glycemic diet

- Low carbohydrate and high-fat diet
- Low-calorie diets
- Weight loss surgery
- Regular exercise in combination with healthy diets

These methods have a similar way of working. They all reduce the daily glucose intake drastically, lower the body's need for insulin, reduce insulin spike in the bloodstream, promote weight loss and prevent weight gain.

2- THE CORTISOL HORMONE

Cortisol is a hormone that is mostly produced in response to stressful situations by the adrenal gland. The hypothalamus, via the pituitary gland, sends a chemical signal to the adrenal glands to produce and release adrenaline and cortisol.

Cortisol is naturally released every day in small and regular quantities. However, like adrenaline, cortisol can also be secreted and released in reaction to physical and emotional stress and triggers the body's fight-or-flight response.

These two stress hormones work simultaneously: adrenaline produces a significant increase in strength, performance, awareness, and increases metabolism. It also lets fat cells release additional energy. Cortisol helps the body make glucose from proteins and increases the body's energy in times of stress quickly.

However, cortisol is also involved in a variety of essential functions for your health. Most of the body cells have cortisol receptors to use this steroid hormone for a variety of critical functions, including:

- blood sugar regulation

- metabolism regulation
- inflammation reduction
- memory formulation

Cortisol is important for your health, but an excess of cortisol can harm your body and induce various undesired symptoms.

WHAT CAUSE HIGH CORTISOL LEVELS?

Several things can cause a high cortisol level, known as Cushing syndrome. This health condition results from your body secreting and releasing too much cortisol.

Cushing syndrome causes many undesired symptoms,

including:

- obesity
- weight gain
- fatty deposits, especially in the face, midsection, and between the shoulders
- purple stretch marks on the arms, breasts, thighs, and abdomen
- thinning skin
- slow-healing injuries

Being under stress induces a constant state of excess cortisol production. And, as seen above, this cortisol drives excess glucose production in a non-fight-or-flight situation. This excess glucose is converted into fat and stored by the body.

Thus, high levels of cortisol increase the risk of obesity highly, induce abdominal obesity, and increase fat storage.

Other factors that cause peaks in cortisol production are carbohydrates deprivation (in a low carb diet, for example) and overconsumption of simple carbohydrates.

In both cases, when blood sugar levels fall, this induces a surge of stress hormones, including cortisol and adrenaline.

STRESS HORMONES AND THEIR ROLE IN THE BODY

Stress hormones are released in reply to body stressors. Hormonal responses of the woman's body to stress are essential, provided they occur less frequently. They may become damaging and unhealthy when they happen too often. Prolonged exposure to porn induces severe damages to the brain and presents evidence that porn is not a healthy stressor.

Stress is habitually accompanied by high energy demand. Consequently, a severe stress situation induces a fast glucose release into the blood, which provides the required energy to deal with the stressful situation.

The principal players in the stress mechanism are:

- The adreno-corticotropic hormone (ACTH),
- The glucocorticoids such as cortisol, adrenaline, and noradrenaline.

When this happens, blood glucose levels rise concurrently with heart rate and blood pressure.

So at its simplest, stress leads to increased blood glucose, high heart rate, and blood pressure, which induces an increased insulin release.

3- THE LEPTIN HORMONE

Leptin is often referred to as the "satiety hormone" because it is produced by fat cells and signals to the brain that the body has enough energy stored and doesn't need to eat more. High levels of leptin lead to a decrease in hunger and an increase in feelings of fullness.

The Leptin hormone was discovered in 1994 and has gained significant interest for its powerful function in weight regulation and obesity. Leptin communicates with specific centers of the brain to influence how the body manages its store of fat. It sends a signal to the brain that the body has enough stored fat, producing the body to burn calories from stored fat and reduce appetite.

Indeed, leptin plays the key regulator of body fat and sends signals to the brain to burn stored fat. This powerful effect would normally prevent obesity, overweight. Early research has seen leptin as the solution for obesity. A supplementation of leptin would induce body fat burning, weight loss, and weight gain prevention. However, experiments revealed an unknown phenomenon that became, until now, not fully understood.

LEPTIN RESISTANCE

Because fat tissues produce leptin, it is released in the bloodstream proportionally to a person's weight. Leptin levels are high for people who are overweight or obese than for people having average weight.

However, research has shown that leptin's benefit in appetite-reducing is very low for obese people, suggesting that people in obesity aren't sensitive to the beneficial effect of leptin and have developed Leptin resistance.

Leptin resistance is an abnormal condition associated with more weight gain for people in overweight or obese. Thus, obese people tend to eat more and more because the hormonal signal that normally sends to the brain that the body has enough stored fat seems to be ignored.

Ongoing research focuses on this kind of leptin resistance in obese people, which stops the brain from acknowledging the leptin's signal.

Some studies, however, suggest that obesity induces multiple cellular processes that attenuate or prevent leptin signaling, amplifying the extent of weight gain. Leptin Resistance may arise from poor leptin transport across the blood-brain barrier (BBB), alteration of the leptin receptor, and defect of leptin signaling...

WAYS TO IMPROVE LEPTIN RESISTANCE AND PROMOTE WEIGHT LOSS

Strong evidence shows that Leptin resistance can be drastically reduced by following these guidelines:

- Eat low-glycemic and moderate-glycemic foods
- Avoid Ultra-processed food: the impact of Ultra-processed food is still under study, but many pieces of evidence suggest that these kinds of foods compromise the integrity of your gut, the normal functioning, and the production of gut hormones.
- Lower your triglycerides: Having high triglycerides levels in your bloodstream can prevent the transport of leptin to your brain.
- Eat healthy protein: Eating healthy proteins can improve leptin sensitivity.
- Eat healthy fats and keep your ratio omega 6/ omega 3 inferior to 3.
- Avoid simple carbohydrates, starches, and eat healthy carbohydrates (complex carbs, fiber).

4- THE GHRELIN HORMONE

Ghrelin, known as the "hunger hormone," is an acyl-peptide responsible for stimulating hunger by sending a chemical signal to tell you when to eat. Ghrelin is secreted and released primarily by the stomach. The small intestine and pancreas also secrete smaller amounts of this hormone.

Ghrelin has various functions. It is known mainly as the hormone that triggers hunger by stimulating the appetite. It induces increases in food intake and promotes fat storage and weight gain.

These findings suggest that by controlling the level of ghrelin and letting it down, we can reduce appetite and food intake.

An experiment consisting of administering ghrelin to people concluded that food intake was increased by 30% in this population.

HOW IS GHRELIN CONTROLLED?

Ghrelin levels are mainly regulated by food intake. Levels of ghrelin in the bloodstream rise typically before eating and when fasting in line with increased hunger.

Experimental studies demonstrated that Ghrelin levels are lower in obese or overweight individuals. Conversely, lean individuals have a high level of ghrelin.

Studies also found that some foods (low-GI foods) slow down the ghrelin released in the bloodstream and thus reduce the impact of hunger hormones.

Soluble and insoluble fibers inhibit ghrelin secretion, implying that eating complex carbohydrates (low-GI and moderate-GI foods) has a positive and significant effect in reducing the production and release of ghrelin.

Glucose also has the same effect as dietary fibers in inhibiting Ghrelin secretion. However, as seen earlier, glucose, starches, and simple carbohydrates must be prohibited due to their impact on rising insulin release.

Recent studies demonstrated that contrary to a common belief, proteins did not reduce the production or release of ghrelin.

5- THE PYY FAMILY

The gut hormone peptide YY 3–36 (PYY3–36) is a polypeptide hormone released from L-cells found in the large intestine and the intestinal mucosa of the ileum.

The hormone PYY is released proportionally to nutrient intake. Indeed, the amount of this hormone is strongly influenced by the number of calories consumed, the macronutrient and micronutrient composition of the eaten meal.

After eating, PYY levels rise within the fifteen first minutes and reach a peak level within ninety minutes. Its primary role is to reduce appetite, the psychological driver for eating. It plays also an important role in regulating the energy balance in the body.

Higher levels of PYY result in reduced appetite reduced calorie intake, and help in weight loss.

Conversely, low levels of PYY induce strong feelings of hunger and cravings while predisposing fatty tissue retention.

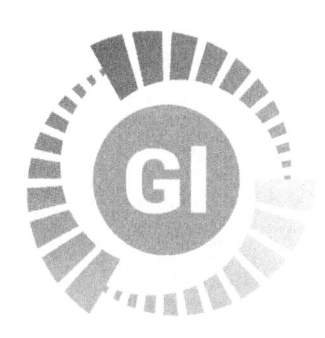

THE GLYCEMIC INDEX DIET

Dr. Jenkins first created the Glycemic Index in the early 1980s to help people with diabetes effectively control and manage their blood glucose levels. The original work involved analyzing 60 foods and measuring how slowly or quickly the foods caused blood sugar levels to rise. The glycemic index is essential to health because high blood sugar spikes can lead to kidney failure or cardiovascular disease. Foods with a low glycemic index release glucose into the blood slowly and evenly. Conversely, foods with a high glycemic index release glucose quickly.

Since this initial work, researchers have found that foods with a low glycemic index (low GI foods) are ideal for weight loss diets and promote weight loss, in addition to their beneficial effects on the pancreas (insulin release), eyes, and kidneys.

The GI is calculated on a scale of 1 to 100. Each food is assigned a score on this scale based on experimental data. A lower score indicates that the food takes a long time to raise blood sugar levels.

Complex carbohydrates are superior to starchy and refined carbohydrates in weight loss and weight gain prevention diets. An excellent way to differentiate healthy carbohydrates is by their glycemic index.

UNDERSTANDING GI VALUES

Glycemic index (GI) values are divided into three categories:

- Low GI: This category includes foods with a GI of less than 55.
- Medium GI: This category includes foods with a GI between 56 and 69.
- High GI: In general, this category should be avoided because the foods cause high spikes in blood sugar levels. They have a GI of 70 or higher.

Comparing GI values can help guide your food choices. For example, muesli has a GI of about 86. A fruit and vegetable smoothie has on a GI of 55.

HOW DOES GLYCEMIC INDEX (GI) DIET WORK?

Eating according to the Glycemic Index Diet looks simple because all you need to know is where different foods fall on the 0 to 100 glycemic index (GI).

- You fill up on low GI foods (GI value: 55 and under)
- Eat smaller amounts of medium GI foods (GI value:56 to 69)
- And mostly avoid high GI foods (GI value: 70 and up)

Lists of foods in the 14 categories are available in this book:

- Beef, Lamb, Veal, Pork & Poultry
- Beverages
- Bread & Bakery Products
- Breakfast Cereals
- Dairy Products & Alternatives
- Soups, Pasta and Noodles
- Fish & Fish Products
- Fruit and Fruit Products
- Legumes and Nuts
- Meat Sandwiches and Ham
- Mixed Meals and Convenience Foods
- Recipe
- Snack Foods and Confectionery
- Vegetables

Besides referring to these lists as needed, there is no difficult weighing or measuring and no need to track your calories intake. However, you will have to concoct your eating plan and menus yourself.

THE GLYCEMIC INDEX AND PORTION SIZES

Since the glycemic load of a food is a function of the glycemic index of the food and the net carbohydrate content of the portion of the food under consideration, it is obvious that the estimated GL will change if you change the portion size. Thus, if you choose a small serving size, you will have a reduced GL, which will result in a reduced sugar intake, regardless of whether the food has a low, moderate, or high glycemic index.

To illustrate this statement, let's consider the fruit watermelon.

Watermelon has a GI of 72 (high). One cup of diced watermelon (152 grams) contains about 11.5 grams of total carbohydrates and 0.5 grams of fiber, which means that watermelon contains about 11 grams of net carbohydrates.

- The glycemic load of watermelon for one cup serving (152 grams) is 7.92, which is equivalent to 7.92 grams of pure glucose.
- The glycemic load of watermelon for a much larger serving (190 grams) is 9.90, which is equivalent to 9.9 grams of pure glucose.
- The glycemic load of watermelon for a much larger serving (240 grams) is 12.50, which is equivalent to 12.5 grams of pure glucose.

The same calculation remains valid and conclusive for foods with a low or moderate glycemic index. As you can see, you can vary the "equivalent" amount of "pure glucose" you consume simply by reducing the portion size. The more you stick to the portion sizes and servings recommended in chapter 10, the more you will get adequate amounts of the nutrients you need to control your diabetes without exceeding the recommended amounts of sugar (50 g in a 2000-calorie diet).

You may be tempted to eat foods with a high glycemic index while reducing your intake. While this may be true on occasion, it would be harmful if done on a regular basis. The GI ranks foods according to the quality of their carbohydrate, and the higher the hyperglycemia induced by the carbohydrate, the higher the associated index. Therefore, favoring low-GI foods is the option of choice for people who want to control their diabetes.

Keep in mind that with the glycemic load approach, you need to add up the GL of all the foods you eat each day and keep your daily GL below 50 for a 2,000-calorie diet. In contrast, what you need to do when following the GI diet is much simpler, you need to check the classification of the food to find out if it is low, moderate or high glycemic, after which you need to choose low glycemic in the first intention and eat the recommended portions. Over time, you will become familiar with the best foods to consume and those to avoid using the Glycemic Index Food Guide in Part II. This is much easier than referring to the GL food chart each time and adding up the GL values of each food you eat.

Chapter 9, Part 1 provides meal planning guidelines with serving sizes for each food group and recommended daily servings. This way, you can rely on the glycemic index without worrying about eating too much sugar. You'll get all the benefits of a low-GI diet without the complex calculations associated with the glycemic load approach.

WILL GLYCEMIC INDEX (GI) DIET HELP YOU LOSE WEIGHT?

Glycemic index diets show much more weight loss in the short and medium term than other diets. Eating foods with a low glycemic index (GI) is the key to weight loss and hormone balance. A 2012 study published in the Journal of the American Medical Association found that low glycemic index (low GI) diets were best and superior at maintaining weight loss when compared to very low carbohydrate diets (such as the ketogenic or keto diet) and low-fat diets. The findings support the GI diet's assertion that "a calorie is not a calorie" and that "different types of foods affect us in different ways, despite having the same number of calories". Another study published in 2014 in The American Journal of Clinical Nutrition supports low glycemic and calorie-restricted diets as more effective than high glycemic and low-fat diets for weight management and weight loss.

2
CARBOHYDRATES, PROTEINS AND FATS: HOW DO MACRONUTRIENTS FIT INTO A HEALTHY LOW-GLYCEMIC DIET?

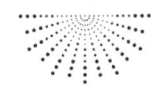

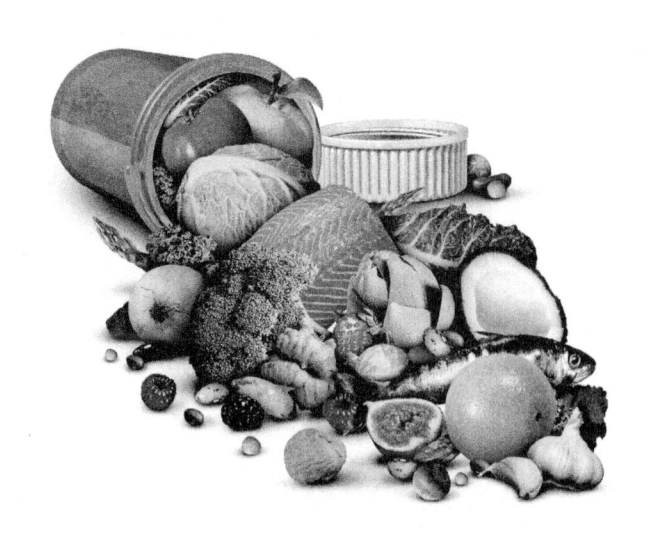

1. Carbohydrates

The choice of high-quality macronutrients is crucial for the success of long-term weight loss or diabetes management.

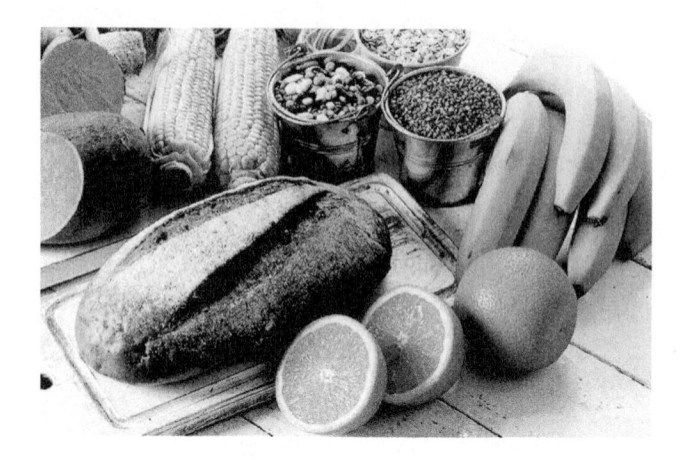

How to make the hormones work for you to lose weight?

Before delving deeper into healthy carbohydrate choices, it is important to note that the following "hormone balancing concepts" must be achieved:

- **Lowering and maintaining insulin levels** will increase your body's insulin sensitivity and reduce any form of insulin resistance.
- **Avoiding spikes in insulin levels**, which are harmful to the pancreas and can cause insulin resistance, as well as cause elevated cortisol levels when blood sugar drops abruptly.
- **Avoiding ultra-processed and highly processed foods** that compromise intestinal integrity and inhibit or reduce the release of leptin, the satiety hormone.
- **Reducing the release of ghrelin, the hunger hormone**, by consuming some nutrients that slow the release of ghrelin into the bloodstream.

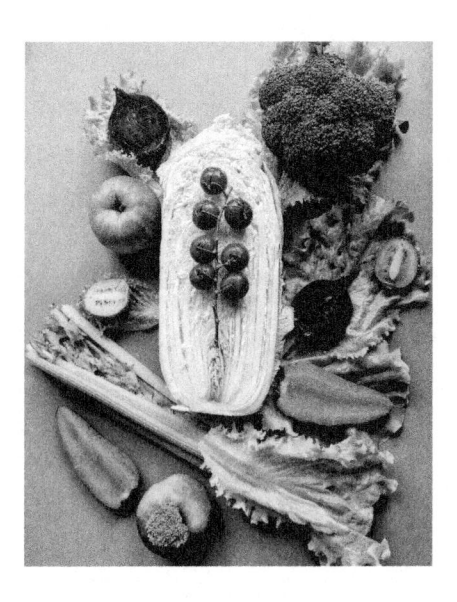

Knowing how carbohydrates can work for you or against you

All carbohydrates, whether they have a low, moderate or high glycemic index, undergo the same metabolic process and break down into blood sugar. Blood glucose levels are critical to the proper functioning of our bodies, but when they spike rapidly and frequently throughout the day, it can be problematic. These spikes occur when we eat mostly high-glycemic foods or large portions of carbohydrate-rich foods with a high glycemic load.

The link between the glycemic index diet, carbohydrates, and weight loss is based on the effect of carbohydrates on blood sugar levels. When you consume high glycemic foods, your blood sugar levels rise quickly and then fall quickly, leading to cravings and hunger, making it difficult to maintain or lose weight. On the other hand, eating low-glycemic foods keeps blood sugar levels stable, which helps reduce cravings and hunger and promotes weight loss.

By following a low-glycemic diet, you can effectively manage your blood sugar levels, leading to weight loss and better weight management. The glycemic index provides a guide to help you make informed food choices, select foods that have a low impact on your blood sugar levels, and keep your metabolism in check.

In addition, following a low-glycemic diet can help control diabetes. People with diabetes often have difficulty managing their blood sugar levels, and a diet focused on low-glycemic foods can help keep these levels in check, reducing the need for insulin or other medications.

Types of Carbohydrates in Your Diet

The primary and main function of carbohydrates is to provide energy to the human body. Dietary carbohydrates can be divided into three major categories:

- Sugars: Short-chain carbs found in foods such as fructose, glucose, sucrose, and galactose.
- Starches: Long-chain of glucose molecules, which get transformed into glucose during digestion.
- Fibers: are divided into soluble and insoluble.

Carbohydrates can also be divided according to their chemical composition into simple and complex carbs:

- Complex carbohydrates are formed by sugar molecules that are linked together in complex and long chains. Complex carbs are found in vegetables, fruits, peas, beans, and whole grains and contain natural fiber. These types of food are healthy.
- Simple carbohydrates are transformed quickly by the body and induce an increased sugar blood level. They are found in high amounts in processed foods and refined sugars. The consumption of this type of carbs is associated with health problems like type 2 diabetes, obesity, metabolism problem. Simple carbs foods are also deprived of essential nutrients and vitamins.

Choosing the best carbohydrates

Achieving your goals in weight loss, weight maintenance, or diabetes management depends on adapting your eating plan to make the insulin, leptin, and ghrelin hormones work for you. *The quality of the carbohydrates you ingest* is crucial in adjusting the level of the hormones, as stated at the beGinning of this chapter. For instance, low-quality carbs (high glycemic foods) are quickly digested and lead to blood sugar spikes, which will play against you and may cause weight gain, obesity, insulin resistance, and increased cortisol levels. Conversely, the soluble and insoluble fibers in whole foods (low glycemic foods) are known to offset glucose conversion, prevent higher insulin supplies, and avoid irregular blood sugar variations that induce an excess of cortisol.

Foods with a low glycemic index are known for their property to release glucose in the blood slowly and regularly. Conversely, Foods that have a high glycemic index are known for their property to release glucose rapidly. Researches suggest that foods with a low glycemic index (LGi foods) are ideal for weight loss diets and foster weight loss, in addition to their positive effect on the pancreas (insulin release), eyes, and kidney.

The glycemic index (Gi) is formed on a scale from 1 to 100. Each food gets a score on this scale according to experimental data. A lower score indicates that food takes a long time to raise blood sugar levels.

---

2. Protein

Protein is one of the three main types of macronutrients found in foods. In a low GI diet, protein is consumed in moderate amounts according to the glycemic index of the food. Eating an adequate amount of protein is extremely important for your health because it plays a crucial role in your body's vital processes and metabolism, such as building and repairing tissues; building muscle, blood, hair, and skin; and producing hormones, enzymes, and other body chemicals.

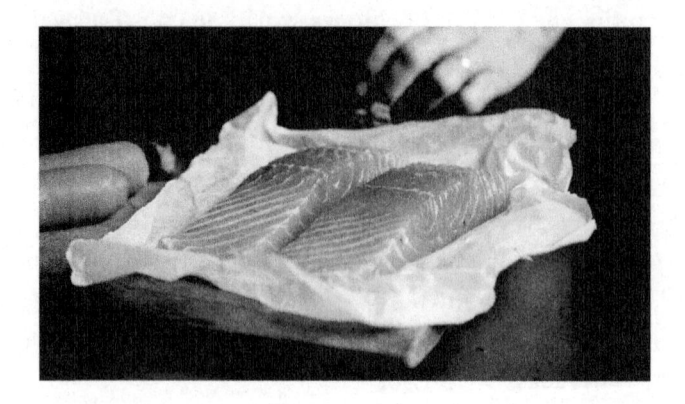

Unlike fats and carbs, the human body does not store protein, and you need to eat the necessary amount to keep the right hormonal balance and a healthy body.

Eating protein reduces levels of ghrelin (the hunger hormone) and stimulates the production of the satiety hormones (PYY and GLP-1)

When you eat protein, it's transformed into amino acids, which help your body with various processes such as building muscle and regulating immune function.

Protein intake and GI diet

In addition to the aforementioned benefits of protein, it also helps with weight loss and weight management. High-protein foods have been shown to have a higher thermic effect, meaning that your body burns more calories digesting protein than it does digesting fats or carbohydrates. In turn, protein helps to increase satiety and satisfaction, leading to a reduction in overall caloric intake.

As part of a low-GI diet, it's important to focus on consuming high-quality protein sources such as lean meats, poultry, fish, eggs, and dairy products, as well as plant-based protein sources such as legumes, nuts, and seeds. The goal is to choose protein-rich foods that are also low on the glycemic index, as high-GI protein sources can still raise blood sugar levels and negatively impact weight loss and blood sugar management.

Protein plays a vital role in overall health and well-being and is an important component of a low-GI diet for weight loss and diabetes management. By including adequate amounts of high-quality protein in your meals, you can help regulate your hormones, build and repair tissue, and promote feelings of fullness and satisfaction.

Guidelines for individualized protein intake

The RDA (international Recommended Dietary Allowance) for protein is 0.8 g per kg of body weight, regardless of age. This recommendation is derived as the minimum amount to maintain nitrogen balance; however, it is not optimized for women's needs or physical activity levels.

Considering different parameters, we recommend a protein intake of 1.4-1.8 grams per kg of your body weight. Going to 1.9 grams per kg of your body weight in the premenstrual phase may be the right choice if you suffer from troubles associated with period approaches (for women).

The Protein Quality

The optimal source of protein is based on the calculation of the PDCAA (Protein Digestibility Corrected Amino Acid) Score or the DIAA (Digestibility Indispensable Amino Acid) Score. Thus, animal-based foods are identified as a superior source of protein because they offer a complete composition of essential amino acids, with higher bioavailability and digestibility (>90%).

Collagen, an essential ingredient

Collagen is the most abundant type of proteins in the human body. Ligaments, tendons, skin, hair, nails, discs, and bones are collagen.

During the normal aging process, your body begins to experience a decline in the synthesis of collagen proteins. According to studies, this decline in collagen production starts around 30, at a rate of 1% per year. At the age of fifty, the rate jump to up to 3%, causing health issues:

- Muscle stiffness
- Aging joint
- Wrinkles and fine lines
- Lack of tone
- Aging skin
- Healing of wounds slower
- Frequent fatigue.

Consuming more collagen will boost your body's collagen protection. So we recommend that your daily intake of collagen represent 25 to 35% of protein.

The beneficial effects include, intestinal health, less articular pain, less hair loss, better skin, increased muscle mass

Foods rich in collagen

Here are some of the best collagen-containing foods you can add to your diet:

Bone broth

Made by simmering bones, tendons, ligaments, and skin of beef, bone broth is an excellent source of collagen, as well as several essential amino acids. Bone broth is also available in powder, bar, or even capsules for a collagen food supplement that is easy to add to your routine.

Spirulina

This kind of seaweed offers an excellent source of plant-based amino acids, which are key components of collagen.

Codfish

Codfish, like most other types of white fish, is a good source of collagen in addition to selenium, vitamin B6 and phosphorus.

Eggs

Eggs are a good source of collagen, including glycine and proline.

Gelatin

Gelatin is one of the best collagen-rich foods available. This is why it is advised to include it in your weight-loss diet.

---

3. Fats

After carbohydrates, it is essential to optimize the choice of your dietary fat.

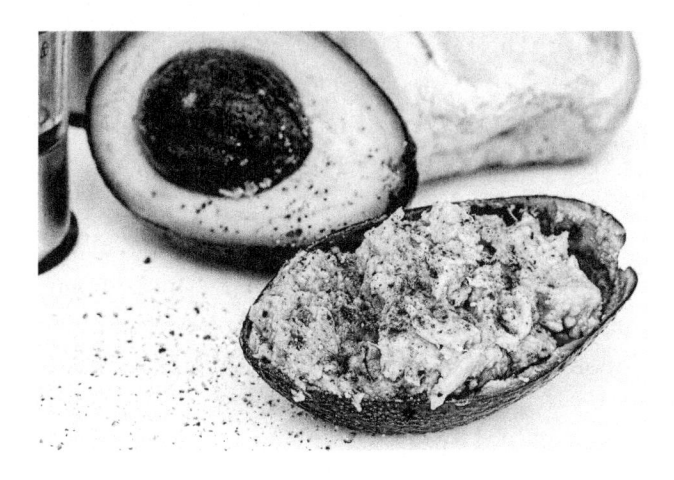

Fat is an essential macronutrient present in food, so you must understand the following information to guide you throughout your diet journey.

What is fat, and why it is essential for your health?

Dietary fats are found in both animals and vegetables and are essential for your living since they provide your body energy and support cell growth.

Fats also provide some valuable benefits and play essential roles, including:

- Help your body absorb some nutrients such as vitamins A, D, E, and K.
- Help your body produce the necessary hormones.
- Regulate inflammation and immunity issues.
- Maintain the health of your body's cells (e.g., skin, hair cells)

How many different fats are there?

There are four main types of fats in foods, based on their chemical structure and physical properties:

- Saturated fat: This type of fat is characterized by having as many hydrogen atoms as possible attached to the fatty acid chain of carbon atoms. While historically considered "bad" for health, recent studies have challenged this perception and suggest a more nuanced view.
- Trans Fat: This form of unsaturated fat is associated with several adverse health effects and should be limited in the diet.
- Monounsaturated fat: This type of unsaturated fat has only one double bond and is associated with beneficial health effects. Foods rich in monounsaturated fat include olive oil, avocados, and some nuts.
- Polyunsaturated fat: This type of unsaturated fat is further divided into omega-3 and omega-6 fatty acids, both of which have beneficial health effects.

What is cholesterol?

Cholesterol is a waxy, fat-like substance found in all the cells in the body and is necessary for the production of various hormones, enzymes, and other body chemicals. Most of the cholesterol in the bloodstream is produced by the liver, not obtained from dietary sources. A balanced level of cholesterol is important for overall health.

What types of fat should you eat?

When it comes to fats in the diet, it's best to focus on eating fats found naturally in food, rather than processed varieties. Some healthy sources of fat include

- Butter and ghee (To be consumed in moderation)
- Cheese (To be consumed in moderation)
- Avocado (the fruit or avocado oil)
- Coconut (meat, cream, oil, milk, butter)
- Cacao butter
- Duck fat (To be consumed in moderation)
- Medium-chained triglyceride (MCT) oil
- Sardines, anchovies
- Salmon
- Olives and olive oil
- Macadamias and macadamia oil
- Almonds, Brazil nuts, hazelnuts, pecans

What are fatty acids?

Fatty acids are a type of hydrocarbon chain consisting of a carboxyl group at one end and a methyl group at the other. The biological activity of fatty acids is determined by the length of the carbon chain and the number and positioning of the double bonds within it.

Saturated fats have no double bonds in the acyl chain, while unsaturated fatty acids contain at least one double bond.

Unsaturated fatty acids with two or more double bonds are known as polyunsaturated fatty acids (PUFAs) and have been associated with cholesterol-lowering properties. The two main families of PUFAs are omega-3 and omega-6.

What are omega-3 fatty acids?

Omega-3 are a class of polyunsaturated fats that the body cannot produce, so it is important to get them from your diet.

There are several types of omega-3 fatty acids that vary in their chemical structure. The three most common types are

- Eicosapentaenoic acid (EPA)
- Docosahexaenoic acid (DHA)
- Alpha-linolenic acid (ALA)

Omega-3 fats play important roles in the body and have been shown to

- Improve heart health
- Support mental health
- Reduce weight and waist size
- Decrease liver fat
- Support infant brain development
- Fight inflammation
- Prevent dementia
- Promote bone health

It is important to include omega-3 fatty acids in a weight loss or anti-inflammatory diet because of their many health benefits for the heart, brain, and metabolism.

What are omega-6 fatty acids?

Omega-6 fatty acids, like omega-3 fatty acids, are polyunsaturated fatty acids.

These fats are primarily used for energy, so it is important to get the right amount from your diet.

Current recommendations suggest a ratio of 4/1 omega-6 to omega-3 or less, meaning that for every 400 milligrams of omega-6, 100 milligrams of omega-3 should be consumed. However, the Western diet often has a much higher ratio, ranging from 10/1 to 50/1.

Why and how is an excess of omega-6 harmful?

The Western diet, including the keto diet, is typically high in omega-6 polyunsaturated fatty acids and has a very high omega-6 to omega-3 ratio. This has been associated with an increased risk of several diseases, including cancer, cardiovascular disease, autoimmune disease, and inflammatory disease.

Conversely, high levels of omega-3 and a low ratio of omega-6 to omega-3 have been associated with health benefits. For example, a ratio of 4:1 has been associated with a 70% reduction in mortality, and a lower ratio in women with breast cancer has been associated with a reduced risk.

This highlights the importance of the omega-6:omega-3 ratio in weight loss and overall health management.

To improve this ratio, it is recommended to eat fatty fish twice a week, eat whole foods, choose dairy products and meat from grass-fed animals, etc.

3

FOOD, WEIGHT LOSS AND DIABETES

Eating to lower blood sugar is not a one-size-fits-all approach. Different people, even twins, can react very differently to the same foods. However, following the glycemic index eating pattern will ensure that you get the most out of its beneficial effects. People who follow this diet more closely have consistently lower blood sugar levels, lower blood pressure, higher LDL cholesterol, lower HDL cholesterol, and lower triglycerides than those who follow other diets. It is considered healthier than modern fad diets (e.g., keto, low-carb, high-fat) because it focuses on eating low-glycemic whole, unprocessed, or minimally processed foods and avoiding high-glycemic foods and pro-inflammatory agents.

- **Diet, Weight Loss, and Diabetes**

For years, hundreds of diets have been created with great promise for weight loss, reducing inflammation, and reversing diabetes. Low-fat diets and low-carbohydrate, high-fat diets have been considered the best way to lose weight, control diabetes, and achieve a healthy weight. However, there is growing and strong evidence that these diets often do not work:

- Low-fat diets tend to replace fat with easily digested carbohydrates.
- Low-carb, high-fat diets neglect the importance of carbohydrates and often replace them with highly processed fatty foods.
- Fad diets often neglect the body's basic need for a balanced diet.

The best diets that work restrict calories to some degree, provide adequate and quality nutrients, eliminate bad foods, and balance hormones that help lower blood sugar, improve blood sugar control, and regulate weight. Diets work in three main ways:

1. getting you to eat sufficient good foods and/or eliminate bad ones
2. making you aware of foods and nutrients you should include in your diet to achieve weight loss, better diabetes control, and prevent complications.
3. changing some of your bad eating habits and the way you view highly processed foods and refined carbohydrates

The best diet for weight loss and/or diabetes control is one that is good for every part of your body, from your kidneys to your heart to your pancreas. It's also a diet you can embrace and live with for a long time. In other words, it's a powerful, nature-based diet that offers flexible eating patterns, makes healthy choices, eliminates unhealthy foods, and doesn't require an extensive (and probably expensive) shopping or supplement list.

A healthy, balanced diet with sufficient and correct nutritional elements is crucial in the fight against diabetes, weight gain and obesity. Both nutrient deficiencies and excesses are associated with disease and poor health. Nutrient excess, especially in highly processed foods, refined carbohydrates, saturated fats, trans fats, sugar-sweetened foods, and sodium, can lead to serious chronic inflammatory diseases such as autoimmune disease, cardiovascular disease, bone disease, diabetes, and obesity. Nutritional deficiencies, on the other hand, can lead to impaired bodily functions, weight loss, fatigue, and conditions associated with vitamin and mineral deficiencies.

One diet that allows for this is a low glycemic index diet. Such a diet—and its many variations—typically include

- Several servings of plant foods (e.g., vegetables, fruits) per day
- Whole and minimally processed foods
- Daily servings of seeds and nuts
- Healthy fats and oils high in omega-3 fatty acids (canola oil, cod liver oil, fatty fish, flaxseed oil, walnut oil, sunflower oil, etc.)
- Lean protein, mainly from fish, poultry and nuts
- Limited amounts of red meat
- Limited amounts of sodium
- Very limited amounts of refined carbohydrates (e.g., white flour, white rice, white sugar, brown sugar, honey, corn syrup)
- Limited alcoholic beverages
- No high glycemic index foods
- No trans fats
- No highly processed foods

- **Dietary carbohydrates and diabetes**

Increased consumption of carbohydrate-containing foods with a higher glycemic index has been shown to cause large spikes in blood sugar and insulin release, making it more difficult to lose weight and control diabetes, and increasing the risk of developing diabetes in healthy people. Conversely, eating carbohydrate-containing foods with a low glycemic index is associated with positive health outcomes and weight loss.

In addition, many studies have shown that the quality of carbohydrates has a significant impact on inflammation, weight gain, insulin resistance, and diabetes complications. Low-quality carbohydrates, such as highly processed foods and refined carbohydrates, are associated with increased inflammation, both acute and chronic, impaired immune response, poor glycemic control, and increased risk of diabetes complications. Conversely, high-quality foods, such as whole or minimally processed foods with a low glycemic index, are associated with sustained weight loss and better health outcomes, including improved glycemic control and reduced acute and chronic inflammation.

- **Dietary fats and diabetes**

The other important nutrient to consider as part of a glycemic index diet for weight loss and diabetes control is fat. Eating the right amount of fat is important whether you are managing diabetes or trying to achieve a healthy weight.

In addition, fats have more calories per gram than protein or carbohydrates. A gram of dietary fat has almost 9 calories, while a gram of carbohydrate has about 4 calories, or protein has about 4 calories. Therefore, you should be aware of portion sizes when eating fats.

Eating healthy fats in the right amount is also important for managing type 1 and type 2 diabetes and lowering the risk of developing some chronic diseases, such as heart disease, stroke, kidney disease, and chronic inflammatory diseases.

Several studies have shown that replacing trans fats, and saturated fats with unsaturated fats (monounsaturated and polyunsaturated) reduces the risk of cardiovascular disease in high-risk populations, including people with diabetes.

In addition, studies have found that replacing trans and saturated fat intake with low glycemic carbohydrates (e.g., whole grains, high-fiber fruits, high-fiber vegetables, and beans) provides cardiovascular benefits without altering glycemic control.

On the other hand, a growing body of evidence has demonstrated how dietary fat intake affects inflammatory status, focusing on the gut microbiome as an important factor in explaining the increase in inflammatory biomarkers and fat intake. Trans fats are associated with several adverse health effects, exacerbating inflammation and triggering diabetes complications. Consuming high amounts of saturated fat increases LDL (bad) cholesterol, which promotes and aggravates inflammation.

The American Diabetes Association recommends replacing saturated and trans fats with healthier choices such as monounsaturated and polyunsaturated fats.

Healthy fats, such as omega-3 fatty acids, have been linked to reduced inflammation and a lower risk of developing some chronic diseases. Several studies have investigated the role of omega-3 fatty acids in combination with metformin to reduce triglyceride levels in diabetic patients with hypertriglyceridemia. Omega-3 fatty acids were found to be effective in significantly reducing triglyceride levels by 20-65%. Omega-3 fatty acids have also been found to improve the effectiveness of statins and thus reduce the risk of cardiovascular disease in diabetic patients with hypertriglyceridemia.

- **The Essential Role of Vitamin D**

It is established that Vitamin D is essential for normal glucose metabolism and improvement of insulin sensitivity. Therefore, vitamin D supplementation appears to promote glucose-mediated insulin secretion allowing vitamin D to play a beneficial role in glucose metabolism by:

1. regulating insulin secretion and promoting the survival of beta-cells, which results in releasing insulin in a tightly regulated manner to maintain blood glucose levels in the adequate range.
2. regulating the calcium flux within beta-cells, which results in improving insulin secretion directly because insulin secretion is a calcium-dependent process. Vitamin D stimulates insulin secretion and benefits beta-cell secretory function when calcium levels are adequate.
3. modulating the adaptive and innate immune responses which result in a preventative effect on autoimmune such as type 1 diabetes. Vitamin D modulates the immune system's response and prevents the destruction of insulin-secreting pancreatic beta-cells, which causes the development of type 1 diabetes.
4. reducing substantially systemic inflammation involved in insulin resistance and the development of type 2 diabetes. Recent investigations have established that vitamin D plays an essential role in modulating the inflammation system by inhibiting the proliferation of pro-inflammatory cells and regulating the production of inflammatory cytokines.
5. improving insulin sensitivity and enhancing pancreatic beta-cell function.

4
FOODS TO INCLUDE IN YOUR LOW GLYCEMIC DIET

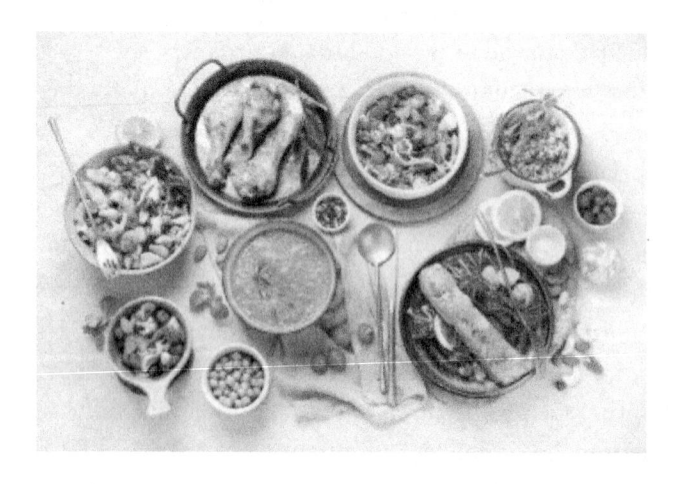

The beneficial effects of an anti-inflammatory diet are due in part to increased consumption of low-glycemic-index vegetables, low-glycemic-index fruits, nuts, olive oil, and low-glycemic whole grains. These foods contain high levels of anti-inflammatory agents that also promote weight loss and diabetes control:

- dietary polyphenols
- flavanoids

- carotenoids
- omega-3 fatty acids
- antioxidants

- **1. Dietary Polyphenols**

There is strong evidence that polyphenol consumption may play a critical role in health by regulating inflammation, metabolism, weight, diabetes, and reducing the risk of developing cardiovascular, neurodegenerative, and cancer diseases.

Dietary polyphenols possess powerful biological properties such as anti-inflammatory, antioxidant, anticarcinogenic, anti-aging, cardiovascular protective, anti-atherosclerotic. The anti-inflammatory effects of polyphenols are well documented and include suppression, inhibition and reduction of any form of inflammation.

Dietary polyphenols are the most prevalent antioxidants in the diet and are ubiquitous in nature. Their sources include vegetables, fruits, legumes, nuts, herbs, seeds, roots, leaves of certain plants, whole grains, curcumin, extra virgin olive oil, dark chocolate, cocoa products, tea, coffee, and red wine. However, they are most abundant in fruits and beverages such as unprocessed fruit juice, tea, coffee, wine, chocolate, cocoa, and beer.

The main dietary polyphenols are:

1. phenolic acids
2. flavonoids
3. stilbenes
4. tannins
5. lignans
6. diferuloylmethane

1.1. PHENOLIC ACIDS SOURCES:

Fruits: blueberry, cranberry, pear, grapefruit, cherry juice, sweet cherry, lemon, peach, orange, apple, apple juice.

Vegetables: potato, lettuce, spinach

Others: tea, coffee, coffee beans, cider

1.3. STILBENES SOURCES

Fruits: grapes, peanuts, strawberry, cranberry

Vegetables: tomato

Others: red wine, white wine, cocoa

1.4. TANNINS SOURCES

Fruits: pomegranate, olive, plum, apple juice, strawberries, raspberries, longan, peach, walnuts, muscadine grape, blackberry, dark grape (seed and skin), white grape (seed and skin),

Vegetables: chickpea, lentils, black-eyed peas

Cereal: haricot bean

Others: cocoa, chocolate, red wine, white wine, coffee, tea, cider, immature fruits

2. FLAVONOIDS

Flavonoids are polyphenolic compounds found in many plants, vegetables, fruits and leaves. Flavanoids have many beneficial health effects due to their potent antioxidant, anti-inflammatory, and anti-carcinogenic activities.

Flavanoids are divided into 7 major subgroups including flavones, flavonols, flavanones, flavanonols, catechins, anthocyanins, and chalcones.

Flavones sources

Fruits: olives, celery

Vegetables: celery hearts, fresh parsley, hot peppers

Spices and herbs: thyme, oregano, dry parsley, rosemary

Flavanols sources

Fruits: apricots, apples, blueberries, cranberries, cherries, blackberries, raspberries, peaches, plums, raisins, grapes, nectarines, pears

Others: green tea, black tea, red wine, white wine, dark chocolate, and cocoa

Flavanones sources

Fruits: lemon, unprocessed lemon juice, unprocessed lime juice, orange, unprocessed orange juice, grapefruit, tangerine, unprocessed tangerine juice

Spices and herbs: peppermint

3. Omega-3 fatty acids

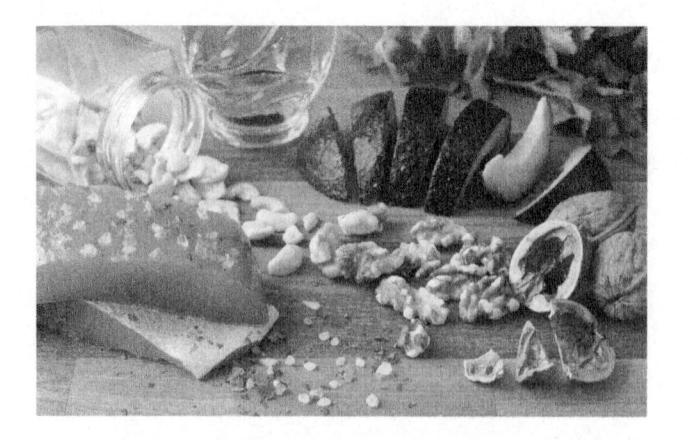

There are four major fats in food, based on their chemical structures and physical properties:

- **3. Olive Oil**

Olive oil is a healthy edible oil made from vegetable fat extracted from the ripe fruit of the olive tree during the crushing process in an oil mill. It is mainly used for raw and cold cooking, but can also be used for frying foods. Olive oil is widely used in cosmetics, pharmaceuticals and soaps.

Extra Virgin Olive Oil (EVOO) is the highest quality olive oil that is completely unprocessed and kept below 75 degrees Fahrenheit during the crushing process.

The beneficial effects of olive oil are well known and documented by various epidemiological studies. Consumption of extra virgin olive oil is associated with better general health, healthy weight and strong anti-inflammatory effects. In fact, extra virgin olive oil contains more than 30 polyphenolic compounds that exert beneficial biological and pharma-nutritional effects on the human body, especially by attenuating pro-inflammatory mediators.

The nutritional composition of virgin olive is comprised of mainly

- monounsaturated fatty acids (69.2% for extra virgin olive oil), mainly Oleic acid (omega-9)
- saturated fats (15.4% for extra virgin olive oil) mainly Stearic acid and Palmitic Acid
- polyunsaturated (9.07% for extra virgin olive oil), mainly Linoleic acid (omega-3)
- Polyphenols
- Vitamin E, Carotenoids, and Squalene

Olive oil has many health benefits including

- reducing inflammation
- protecting against oxidative damage
- offering some potential benefits for weight loss
- treating and preventing arterial hypertension
- Improving blood sugar control
- lowering LDL cholesterol (bad)
- reducing the risk of some cancers
- enhancing digestion and absorption of nutrients

The anti-inflammatory benefits of EVOO increase with daily consumption. A minimum of four tablespoons of extra virgin olive oil per day is required to provide beneficial anti-inflammatory and antioxidant effects.

5

EATING LOW GLYCEMIC AND ANTI-INFLAMMATORY FOODS

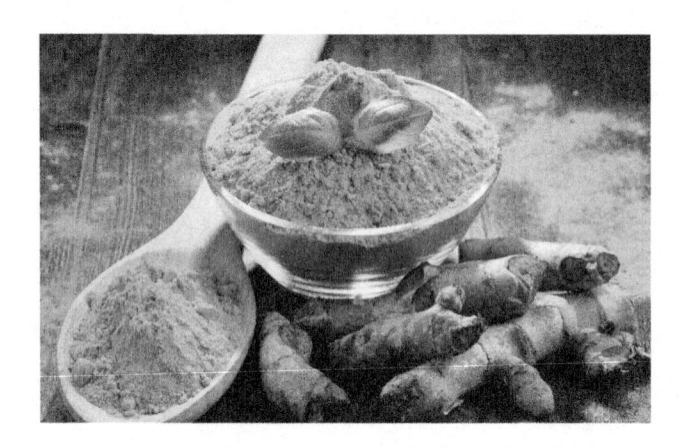

- **1. Eating low glycemic index vegetables and fruits**

In the glycemic index diet, you have to eat low glycemic index fruits and vegetables to keep close control of your blood sugar level, avoid blood sugar spikes that in turn may result in insulin resistance, and weight gain. In addition, non-starchy vegetables and fruits are good sources of anti-inflammatory nutrients such as polyphenols, antioxidants, and flavonoids which contribute to lowering inflammation and, in turn, reducing the risk of diabetes complications.

The serving sizes for low glycemic index vegetables and fruits are equivalent to:

- 1 cup raw or salad vegetables
- 1/2 cup cooked vegetables
- 3/4 cup (6oz) vegetable juice homemade and unsweetened
- ½ cup of cooked beans, lentils, and peas
- 1 medium piece of fruit
- 1 cup (6 oz) of sliced fruits
- ½ cup (4 oz) of fruit juice

The total vegetable intake (per day) is equivalent to 8-10 servings. You have to vary your meals using the maximal recommended amount as follows:

- "Dark-Green Vegetables" group up to 2 servings
- "Red & Orange Vegetables" group up to 3 servings
- "Beans, Peas, Lentils" group up to 2 servings
- "Starchy Vegetables" group up to 1 serving
- "Other Vegetables" group up to 3 servings

The total fruit intake is equivalent to 2-4 servings per day.

- **2. Increasing your Omega-3 Fatty Acids intake**

Omega-3 fatty acids are healthy types of polyunsaturated fats associated with beneficial health effects such as

- decreasing inflammation
- improving heart health

- supporting mental health
- decreasing liver fat
- helping in the prevention of many chronic conditions
- promoting bone health

Strategies to increase your weekly intake of omega-3 fatty acids include regularly eating omega-3-rich nuts and seeds—such as chia seed, flaxseed, Hemp seed—, eating fatty fish—such as salmon, sardines, anchovies, mackerel, and herring. The weekly fish intake is equivalent to 10 servings (a serving is equal to 3 to 4 ounces). So target eating 6-8 servings of fatty fish per week.

- **3. Choosing healthy fats**

The glycemic index diet is rich in omega-3 and lower in omega-6 than most diets. High levels of omega-3 combined with a low (omega-6/omega-3) are associated with many health benefits, including a significant reduction of unnecessary inflammation and diabetes complications. For example, a ratio (omega-6/omega-3) of 4/1 was correlated to a 70% reduction in mortality. So, based on recent studies, you have to keep the ratio (omega-6/omega-3) in the range of 1/1 and 4/1, which is associated with positive health outcomes.

Strategies to achieve an adequate ratio (omega-6/omega-3) include

- consuming fatty fish (e.g., sardines, mackerels, salmon, herring, anchovies) twice a week,
- consuming nuts and seeds (e.g., flax seeds, chia seeds, walnuts) twice a week.

- **4. Increasing olive oil consumption**

Recent studies have established that an extra virgin olive oil-rich diet reduces glucose levels, LDL cholesterol (bad), and triglycerides. In addition, extra virgin olive oil was found to provide potential benefits for weight loss, diabetes prevention, and management.

The anti-diabetes benefits of Extra Virgin Olive Oil (EVOO) increase with the daily ingested amount. A minimum of extra virgin olive oil of four tablespoons per day is necessary to provide beneficial anti-diabetes and antioxidant effects. When cooking, EVOO is an excellent choice as it has been well established that it helps reduce blood sugar levels, reduce blood pressure, lower bad cholesterol (LDL), and decrease inflammation. The nutritional composition of virgin olive is comprised mainly of

- monounsaturated fatty acids (69.2% for extra virgin olive oil), mainly Oleic acid (omega-9)
- saturated fats (15.4% for extra virgin olive oil) mainly Stearic acid and Palmitic Acid
- polyunsaturated (9.07% for extra virgin olive oil), mainly Linoleic acid (omega-3)
- Polyphenols
- Vitamin E, Carotenoids, and Squalene

Strategies to increase your daily intake of olive oil include

- replacing butter with EVOO,
- using olive oil as finishing oil for your meals,
- replacing the oil you use for cooking,
- roasting, and frying with EVOO.

- **5. Including anti-inflammatory spices in your eating plan**

Over the several last decades, extensive research has revealed that some spices and their active components exhibit tremendous anti-inflammatory benefits. Thus, spices have been found to prevent or decrease the severity of diabetes complications as well as a number of chronic conditions such as arthritis, asthma, multiple sclerosis, cardiovascular diseases, lupus, cancer, and neurodegenerative diseases. The most common spices used for their anti-inflammatory activities are

- turmeric,
- green tea,
- garlic,
- ginger,
- cayenne pepper,
- black pepper,
- black cumin,
- clove,
- cumin,
- ginseng,
- cardamom,
- parsley
- cinnamon,
- rosemary,
- chives,
- basil,
- cilantro

In addition, spices have a unique property to add flavor to any meal without adding fats or salt. Therefore, you should consider integrating herbs as part of your daily diet when cooking.

Some strategies for getting more herbs and spices in your diet include

- using some fresh herbs as the main ingredient (e.g., herb salad, tabbouleh salad),
- replacing some green vegetables in salads with herbs,

- substituting (or reducing) salt in a recipe with spices,
- replacing mayonnaise with basil-olive oil preparation,
- drinking 3–4 cups of green tea daily.

- **6. Drinking more water**

Water is critical for life. Without water, there is no life. All of the organs of our body, such as the heart, brain, lungs, and muscles, contain a significant quantity of water and need water to stay healthy.

Every day we lose water, and we need to replace it through a regular water supply. Otherwise, we can suffer from dehydration, which may alter the normal body's functions.

The recommended water intake for men aged 19+ is 3 liters (13 cups), and for women aged 19+ is 2.2 liters (9 cups) each day.

6
AVOIDING HIGH GLYCEMIC AND INFLAMMATORY FOODS

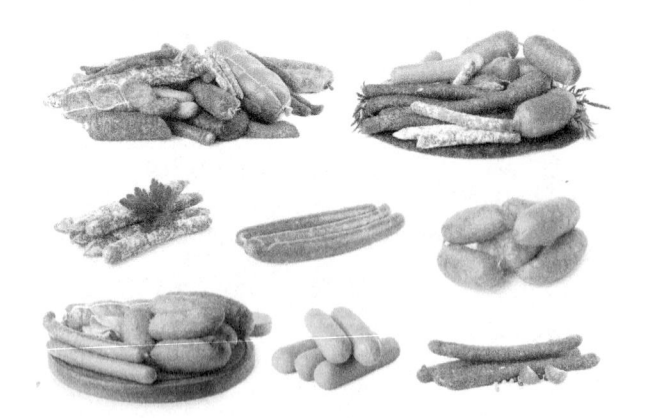

- **1. Limiting moderate glycemic index foods and avoiding high glycemic foods**

Eating according to the Glycemic Index Diet looks simple because all you need to know is where different foods fall on the 0 to 100 glycemic index (GI).

THE ESSENTIAL FOODS LISTS FOR THE GLYCEMIC INDEX DIET

- You fill up on low glycemic index foods (GI value: 55 and under)
- Eat smaller amounts of moderate glycemic index foods (GI value:56 to 69)
- And mostly avoid high glycemic index foods (GI value: 70 and up)

Tables of foods with their glycemic index divided into the 14 categories are available in part II, "Glycemic Index Counter":

- Beef, Lamb, Veal, Pork & Poultry
- Beverages
- Bread & Bakery Products
- Breakfast Cereals
- Dairy Products & Alternatives
- Soups, Pasta, and Noodles
- Fish & Fish Products
- Fruit and Fruit Products
- Legumes and Nuts
- Meat Sandwiches and Ham
- Mixed Meals and Convenience Foods
- Recipe
- Snack Foods and Confectionery
- Vegetables

- **2. Excluding Trans-Fats containing Foods**

Trans-fatty acids are mostly industrially manufactured fats produced during the hydrogenation process that adds hydrogen to liquid vegetable oils to transform the liquid to a solid form at room temperature. Trans fats provide foods with a desirable taste and texture. However, unlike other dietary fats, consuming trans-fatty acids raises the level of your bad cholesterol (LDL), lowers your good cholesterol

(HDL) levels, increases your risk of developing severe cardiovascular conditions certain cancers, and aggravates inflammation. Trans fats may be present in several food products, including:

- fried fast foods, including french fries, fried chicken, battered fish, mozzarella sticks, and doughnuts
- margarine
- peanut butter
- baked goods, such as cakes, pies, and cookies made with margarine or vegetable shortening
- vegetable shortening

Strategies to reduce drastically trans fats intake include

- avoiding or reducing intake of fried fast foods—including french fries, fried chicken, battered fish, mozzarella sticks, and doughnuts—margarine, peanut butter, frozen pizza, baked goods made with margarine or vegetable shortening
- eating smaller portion sizes
- consuming trans-fat-containing foods less frequently.

- **3. Eating a little less red meat but enough proteins**

There is little evidence that red meat may contribute to inflammation and alter glycemic control, while some recent studies revealed that unprocessed red meat might be associated with less inflammation and is safe for people with diabetes or pre-diabetes. However, there is a consensus about the danger of consuming processed red meat such as sausage, bacon, salami, and hot dogs. A 2012 study funded and supported by some health and nutrition government agencies has established the link between processed red meal consumption and increased total mortality. It also revealed that daily unprocessed red meat consumption raised the risk of total mortality by 13%. The study revealed that replacing one serving of red meat per day with other proteins sources such as fish, poultry, and nuts could decrease the risk of mortality by 7-19%.

These findings suggest that you should restrict your red meat intake to reduce inflammation, and prevent diabetes.

Eating an adequate amount of protein is extremely important for your health because proteins play a crucial role in your body's vital processes and metabolisms, such as building and repairing tissues, building muscles, blood, hair, and skin, regulating some inflammatory responses, and producing hormones, enzymes, and other body chemicals. The weekly recommended proteins intake is equivalent to

- 30 servings of animal proteins (mainly lean white meat, and eggs)
- 10 servings of seafood
- 5 servings of nuts and seeds

By restricting red meat intake in the range of 1/5 to 1/4 of animal proteins (e.g., 6 to 7.5 servings of red meat per week), you may experience improvement in your overall health and reduction of some symptoms caused by inflammation.

7
EATING WHOLE AND MINIMALLY PROCESSED FOODS

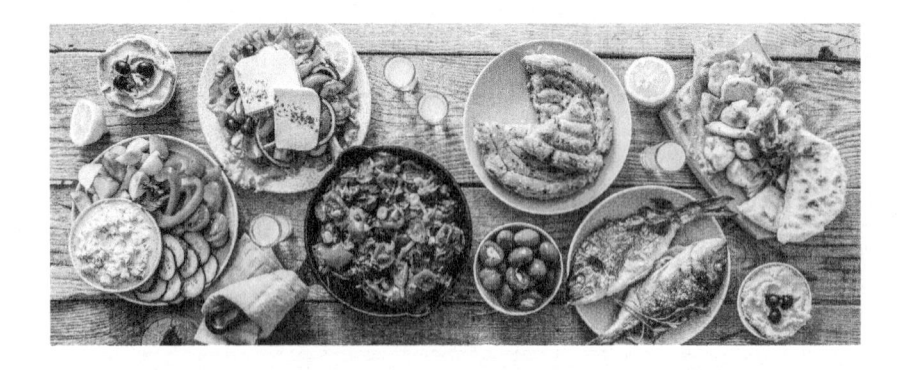

Most Americans don't eat whole foods anymore. They eat processed and highly-processed foods that are generally inferior to unprocessed or minimally processed foods. In fact, highly-processed foods are generally industrially-made and contain many ingredients, including high-fructose corn syrup, trans fats, monosodium glutamate, artificial sweeteners, flavors, colors, and other chemical additives. Highly-processed foods are believed to be a significant contributor to the obesity epidemic in the world, promoting diabetes, chronic inflammation, and the prevalence of autoimmune diseases. Therefore, we must distinguish between healthy processed foods to include in the glycemic index diet for weight loss and diabetes control and those to exclude because they are considered unhealthy and pro-inflammatory. For this reason, the next chapter (chapter 10) is fundamental because it contains foods groups based on the NOVA classification system. To adhere to the glycemic index diet for weight loss and diabetes control, you must get familiar with the four NOVA foods groups.

Whole food refers to unprocessed or minimally processed food— a nature-made food without added sugars, fat, sodium, flavorings, or other artificial ingredients. It has not been broken down by the man's intervention into its components and refined into a new form. Whole Foods are generally close to their natural state, unprocessed, and unrefined. Whole foods have little to no additives or preservatives.

A glycemic index diet for weight loss and diabetes control is not a specific diet. Instead, it refers to an eating plan that primarily selects low glycemic and whole foods and provides many health benefits, including better glycemic control, diabetes complication prevention, inflammation reduction, and hypertension prevention and treatment.

- **The glycemic index diet for weight loss and diabetes control — Main Principles**

The glycemic index diet for weight loss and diabetes control is a revolutionary balanced, easy, long-term, and sustainable diet that selects low glycemic whole, minimally processed foods and limits animal products. It mainly focuses on plants, including vegetables, fruits, whole grains, legumes, seeds, and nuts, which should make up most of what you eat. You then have to design your eating plan around **unprocessed and minimally processed foods (NOVA group 1 of foods)** and, as much as you can, **avoid those that are processed**

(NOVA group 2 of foods) and **absolutely exclude highly processed (NOVA group 3 of foods)**.

The glycemic index diet for weight loss and diabetes control supplies your body with low glycemic unprocessed or minimally processed foods **(NOVA group 1 of foods)**, with little to no unhealthy added constituents. You don't have to focus on calorie, protein, fat, or carb counting. Instead, you have to concentrate on eating foods that do not cause high blood sugar spikes and battle inflammation.

The importance of glycemic index component is critical because one can adopt a whole foods diet and still end up eating unhealthy carbohydrates-containing foods or fatty foods. Merely avoiding processed and refined foods is not the answer to better glycemic control, diabetes complications prevention, and inflammation reduction. Frequently eating carbohydrates-containing foods that cause high spikes in your blood sugar may make it harder to control your blood sugar and put you at increased risk of diabetes complications.

Coconut, coconut oil, palm kernel oil, and palm oil are fall in the category of whole foods but are full of saturated fats. Many experts, including the American Diabetes Association, the American Heart Association, claim that replacing foods high in saturated fat with healthier alternatives may lower LDL cholesterol and triglycerides in the blood. In addition, oils rich in saturated fats are associated with increased inflammation and chronic diseases.

Thus the glycemic index component is critical to addressing such problems and providing a robust solution to achieve a healthy weight or win against diabetes.

\

8

12 PRINCIPLES & TIPS OF LOW-GLYCEMIC EATING

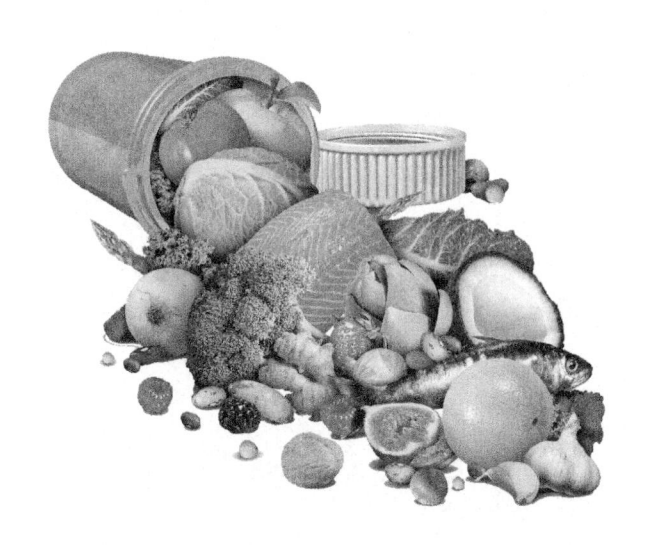

Healthy weight loss

Losing weight very quickly may not be the best option.

People who are successful at keeping weight off lose weight progressively and regularly (about 1 to 2 pounds per week).

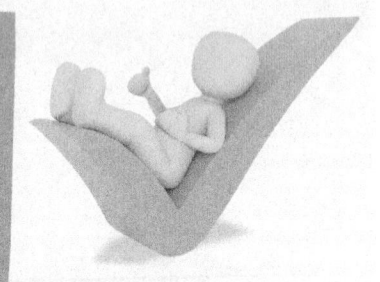

Tips

Do not ban any foods from your GI weight loss plan, especially the ones you like. Instead mix them with low GI food to lower the overall GI

Facts

Healthy weight loss isn't just about following a low-glycemic diet but about a continuous lifestyle, including lasting changes in your daily eating and exercise practice.

Risks

Losing weight too fast could put you at risk of developing many health problems, including decrease in metabolism, hormonal imbalance, muscle loss, nutritional deficiencies

The caloric deficit

The caloric deficit is an important principle to achieve your weight loss goal.

Keep in mind that calories are not equal, and choose high-quality food by following the guidelines in this chapter.

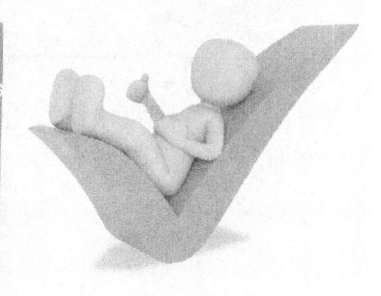

Tips

The first thing you have to do before starting the low glycemic diet is to figure out how much you need to lose.

Facts

Always remember that even small losses in weight can drive better health and sustainable weight loss.

Risks

You need to eat a minimum amount of calories to maintain a healthy metabolism:
- 300 calories for breakfast,
- and 500 calories each for lunch and dinner

Dietary fiber in GI

Fiber plays a crucial role in weight loss management, weight maintenance, diabetes management and obesity control.

Fiber plays a crucial role in weight loss management because it slows down the absorption of sugars, and digestion takes longer.

Tips

Raw fruit and vegetable are lower in glycemic index than juices, for example.

Benefits

Eating a low glycemic diet implies choosing foods with high fiber content in place of low-fiber foods, provided their glycemic index is low to moderate.

Facts

Dietary fiber comprises many essential molecules, including cellulose, dextrins, lignin, pectins, inulin, chitins, waxes, beta-glucans, and oligosaccharides. the higher dietary fibre content frequently associated with low-GI foods may add to the metabolic merits of a low-GI diet.

THE ESSENTIAL FOODS LISTS FOR THE GLYCEMIC INDEX DIET

Unprocessed foods

Unprocessed foods are more complex to digest than processed foods, so they are generally low glycemic index.

Keep in mind that calories are not equal, and choose high-quality food by following the guidelines in this chapter.

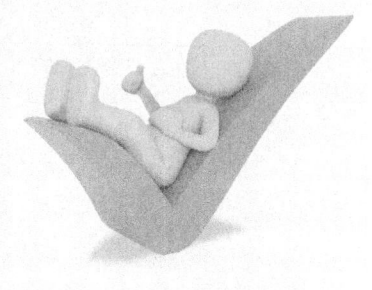

Tips

Eating a low glycemic diet implies choosing unprocessed foods in place of processed alternatives.

Facts

Studies show that the proportion of carbohydrates digested was significantly higher for processed foods than the unprocessed cooked foods, which produced a higher glycemic index.

Risks

processed foods are always suggested to be a great contributor to the obesity epidemic and rising prevalence of chronic diseases like inflammations, heart disease and type 2 diabetes

Fat in low GI diet

All kinds of fats lower the glycemic response of carbohydrates.

White bread with butter is harder to digest than white bread, so that you can reduce the glycemic index of foods using such a trick.

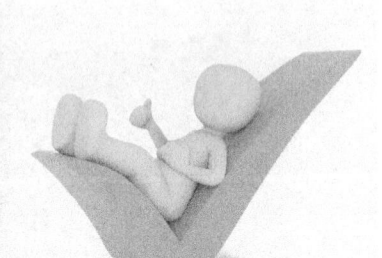

Tips

The first thing you have to do before starting the low glycemic diet is to figure out how much you need to lose.

Facts

When following the low glycemic index diet, it is essential to keep in mind that high-GI foods are not entirely banned. When eaten with fats, protein foods, or low-GI foods, or cooked firmly (like al dente for pasta) the overall GI value of the meal would be about low to medium.

Benefit

It is admitted that adding fat and protein to high-carbohydrate food content reduces glycemic responses by delaying gastric emptying and stimulating insulin secretion.

Cooking time in GI

Longer cooking time makes some foods easier to digest, increasing the blood sugar level.

Keep in mind that calories are not equal, and choose high-quality food by following the guidelines in this chapter.

Tips

When eating a low glycemic index diet, it is essential to remember that high-GI foods are not entirely banned.

Facts

When cooked al dente, pasta is more complex to digest than overcooked one. It has a lower glycemic index—reducing cooking time and eating foods while still firm means difficult digestion and smooth insulin release in the bloodstream.

Benefits

When eaten cooked firmly (like al dente for pasta), the new GI value of the meal would be about low to medium.

Protein in GI diet

Proteins slow the digestion of carbohydrates and lower the effects of high-glycemic-index food on your blood sugar.

Protein plays a crucial role in vital processes and metabolism of your body, such as building and repairing tissues, building muscles, blood, hair, and skin, and producing hormones, enzymes, and other body chemicals.

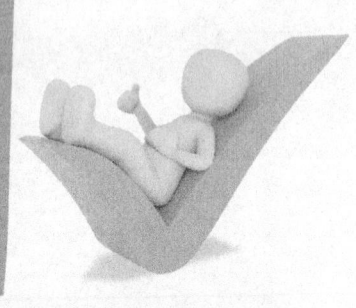

Tips

Eggs have a relatively low glycemic index and are perfect. So if you eat a boiled egg with your whole wheat bread or white bread toast, your meal will have a lower GI.

Benefits

You can eat high-glycemic index foods provided you combine them with low-glycemic index foods like eggs, olive oil, and butter.
The RDA (International Recommended Dietary Allowance) for protein is 0.8 g per kg of body weight, regardless of age.

Facts

The study "Egg ingestion in adults with type 2 diabetes" published in 2016 by a group of researchers showed that the daily inclusion of eggs in the habitual eating plan for 12 weeks reduced body weight, visceral fat rating, waist circumference, and percent body fat in adults with type 2 diabetes.

THE ESSENTIAL FOODS LISTS FOR THE GLYCEMIC INDEX DIET

High GI Foods

Eating a low glycemic diet implies replacing high glycemic index foods with low glycemic index and moderate glycemic index alternatives.

When eating a low glycemic index diet, it is essential to remember that high-GI foods are not entirely banned.

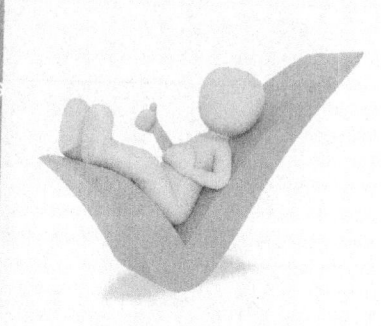

Tips

You can lower the negative impact of foods with a high glycemic index by combining them with low glycemic index foods.

Benefits

If you want to eat a white-bread bagel, for example, try adding a boiled egg or spreading it with a tablespoon of olive oil, butter, or peanut butter instead of jams or strawberry jelly.

Facts

Always remember that even small losses in weight can drive better health and sustainable weight loss.

Acidic drinks & foods

Foods that are considered acidic generally have a pH level of 4.6 or lower.

Keep in mind that although these foods have positive impact in GI, their initial acidity could worsen symptoms for those with upper gastrointestinal issues like an ulcer or reflux.

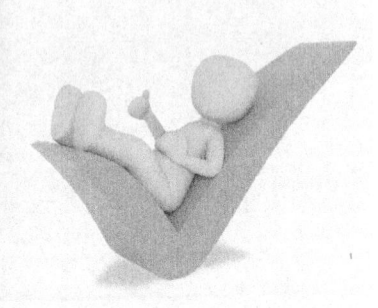

Tips

Adding Citrus fruits like lemons to meals with a high-glycemic index helps lower the meal's overall glycemic index.

Benefits

The addition of vinegar to starches-rich meals with a high-glycemic-index character reduces the meal's glycemic index and increases the post-meal satiety.

Facts

Many studies have reported the remarkable effect of acidic drinks and foods in reducing the glycemic response to carbohydrates-rich meals by 20 to 50%.

THE ESSENTIAL FOODS LISTS FOR THE GLYCEMIC INDEX DIET

Omega-3 & GI diet

Omega-3 fatty acids are a type of polyunsaturated fats classified as "essential fats

Keep in mind that calories are not equal, and choose high-quality food by following the guidelines in this chapter.

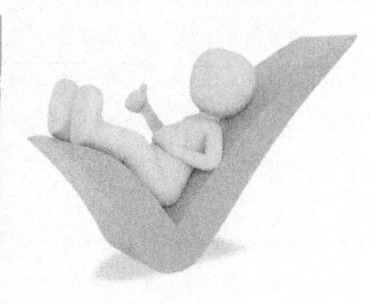

Tips

The best way to ensure optimal omega-3 consumption is to eat fatty fish at least twice per week. However, if you don't eat fatty fish or seafood, you may consider taking a supplement.

Facts

The omega-3 fatty acids have several potential health benefits, including supporting a weight loss diet. Fish oil omega-3s will help you lose inches and shed body fat. The USDA Food Guide Pyramid recommends between 1 and 3 grams of omega-3 per day.

Benefits

Omega-3 is an essential fat that you must integrate into your low-glycemic diet. They have significant benefits for your heart, brain, and metabolism.

Omega-6 in GI diet

Omega-6 fats from vegetable oils and other sources are good for the heart and body.

Good sources of omega-6 include : Safflower oil, sunflower oil, corn oil, soybean oil, sunflower seeds, walnuts, pumpkin seeds.

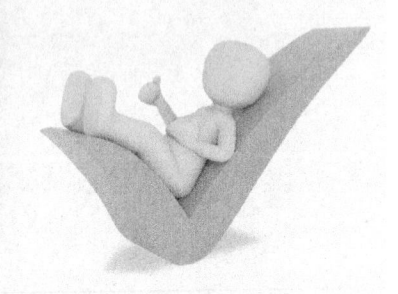

Tips

The first thing you have to do before starting the low glycemic diet is to figure out how much you need to lose.

Benefits

Following different recommendations and guidelines, we recommend a ratio of 4/1 omega-6 to omega-3 or less, which means that for 400 milligrams of omega-6, you have to consume 100 milligrams of omega-3.

Facts

Unlike saturated and trans fats, the polyunsaturated omega-3 and omega-6 fats and the monounsaturated fats are healthy, if consumed moderately.

Collagen & GI diet

The most abundant type of protein in your body is collagen.

Keep in mind that calories are not equal, and choose high-quality food by following the guidelines in this chapter.

Tips

Ligaments, tendons, skin, hair, nails, discs, and bones are collagen. Eating collagen will positively impact them.

Benefits

Consuming more collagen will boost your body's collagen protection. So we recommend that your daily intake of collagen represents 25 to 35% of protein.

Facts

During the normal aging process, the body begins to experience a decline in the synthesis of collagen proteins around 30, at a rate of 1% per year. At the age of fifty, the rate jump to up to 3%, causing health issues: muscle stiffness, aching joints, wrinkles, and fine lines; lack of tone, sagging skin, healing of wounds slower, frequent fatigue.

9
MEAL PLANNING GUIDELINES

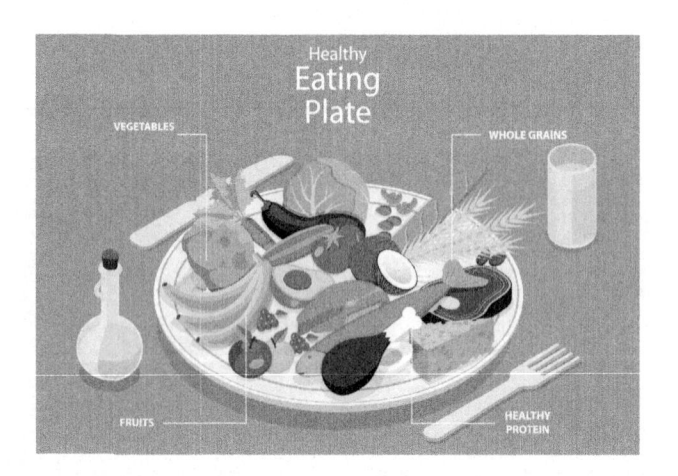

The glycemic index dietary guidelines ensure that recommendations for a successful low-glycemic diet are met. Instead of giving strict recommendations, it gives options in each food group you can choose from. Each food has anti-inflammatory properties and a low glycemic index.

All foods are assumed to be

THE ESSENTIAL FOODS LISTS FOR THE GLYCEMIC INDEX DIET

- unprocessed or minimally processed (NOVA group 1 of Food (please refer to part III for more details)),
- in nutrient-dense forms
- lean or low-fat
- prepared and cooked with minimal added sugars, salt (sodium), refined carbohydrates, saturated fat, or trans fats.

The number of daily calories depends on your personal needs. You have to eat a balanced diet daily by following the general guidelines in this chapter and the amounts of food from each food group required to meet the low-glycemic diet goals. Recommended amounts of foods in each food group are given to allow you to design your weekly and monthly eating plan.

1- Vegetables

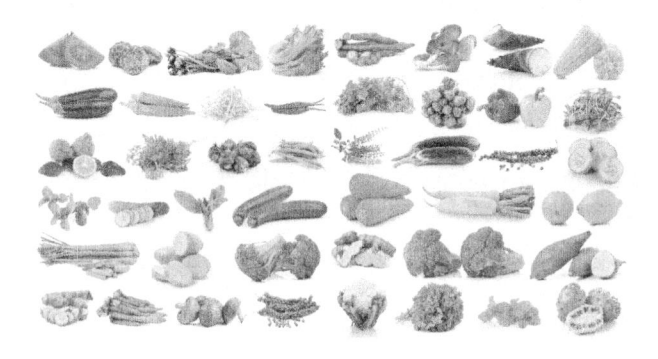

1.1 WHAT IS THE PORTION SIZE?

The standard serving sizes for vegetables and vegetable juices are equivalent to:

- 1 cup raw or salad vegetables
- 1/2 cup cooked vegetables

- 3/4 cup (6oz) vegetable juice homemade and unsweetened
- ½ cup of cooked beans, lentils, and peas

All vegetables in this list are low-glycemic-index and anti-inflammatory

How Much a Day?

Total vegetable intake: up to 10 servings

- "Dark-Green Vegetables" group up to 2 servings
- "Red & Orange Vegetables" group up to 3 servings
- "Beans, Peas, Lentils" group up to 2 servings
- "Starchy Vegetables" group up to 3 servings
- "Other Vegetables" group up to 3 servings

For most people, following the low-glycemic diet will require an increase in total vegetable intake from all five vegetable subgroups ("Dark-Green Vegetables", "Red & Orange Vegetables", "Beans, Peas, Lentils", "Starchy Vegetables", "Other Vegetables").

Strategies to increase total vegetable intake include

1. increasing the vegetable content of mixed dishes (more vegetables)
2. adding vegetables to breakfast
3. blending and consuming vegetables into smoothies
4. preparing sauces with vegetables
5. consuming regularly vegetable-based soups

1.2 Dark-Green Vegetables:

THE ESSENTIAL FOODS LISTS FOR THE GLYCEMIC INDEX DIET

- **amaranth leaves** (all fresh, frozen, cooked, or raw)
- **arugula (rocket)** (all fresh, frozen, cooked, or raw)
- **bok choy (Chinese chard)** (all fresh, frozen, cooked, or raw)
- **dandelion greens** (all fresh, frozen, cooked, or raw)
- **kale** (all fresh, frozen, cooked, or raw)
- **mustard greens** (all fresh, frozen, cooked, or raw)
- **rapini (broccoli raab)** (all fresh, frozen, cooked, or raw)
- **swiss chard** (all fresh, frozen, cooked, or raw)
- **turnip greens** (all fresh, frozen, cooked, or raw)
- **broccoli** (all fresh, frozen, cooked, or raw)
- **chamnamul** (all fresh, frozen, cooked, or raw)
- **chard** (all fresh, frozen, cooked, or raw)
- **collards** (all fresh, frozen, cooked, or raw)
- **poke greens** (all fresh, frozen, cooked, or raw)
- **romaine lettuce** (all fresh, frozen, cooked, or raw)
- **spinach** (all fresh, frozen, cooked, or raw)
- **taro leaves** (all fresh, frozen, cooked, or raw)
- **watercress** (all fresh, frozen, cooked, or raw)

1.3 Red and Orange Vegetables

- **acorn squash** (all fresh, frozen, vegetables or juice, cooked or raw)
- **butternut squash** (all fresh, frozen, vegetables or juice, cooked or raw)
- **calabaza** (all fresh, frozen, vegetables or juice, cooked or raw)
- **carrots** (all fresh, frozen, vegetables or juice, cooked or raw)
- **red bell peppers** (all fresh, frozen, vegetables or juice, cooked or raw)
- **hubbard squash** (all fresh, frozen, vegetables or juice, cooked or raw)
- **orange bell peppers** (all fresh, frozen, vegetables or juice, cooked or raw)

- **sweet potatoes** (all fresh, frozen, vegetables or juice, cooked or raw)
- **tomatoes** (all fresh, frozen, vegetables or juice, cooked or raw)
- **pumpkin** (all fresh, frozen, vegetables or juice, cooked or raw)
- **winter squash** (all fresh, frozen, vegetables or juice, cooked or raw)

1.4 Beans, Peas, Lentils

- **beans** (all cooked from dry)
- **peas** (all cooked from dry)
- **chickpeas (Garbanzo Beans)** (all cooked from dry)
- **lentils** (all cooked from dry)
- **black beans** (all cooked from dry)
- **black-eyed peas** (all cooked from dry)
- **Bayo beans** (all cooked from dry)
- **cannellini beans** (all cooked from dry)
- **great northern beans** (all cooked from dry)
- **edamame** (all cooked from dry)
- **kidney beans** (all cooked from dry)
- **lentils** (all cooked from dry)
- **lima beans** (all cooked from dry)
- **mung beans** (all cooked from dry)
- **pigeon peas** (all cooked from dry)
- **pinto beans** (all cooked from dry)
- **split peas** (all cooked from dry)

1.5 Starchy Vegetables

- **breadfruit** (all fresh, or frozen)
- **burdock root** (all fresh, or frozen)

- **cassava** (all fresh, or frozen)
- **jicama** (all fresh, or frozen)
- **lotus root** (all fresh, or frozen)
- **plantains** (all fresh, or frozen)
- **salsify** (all fresh, or frozen)
- **taro root (dasheen or yautia)** (all fresh, or frozen)
- **water chestnuts** (all fresh, or frozen)
- **yam** (all fresh, or frozen)
- **yucca** (all fresh, or frozen)

1.6 Other Vegetables

- **asparagus** (all fresh, frozen, cooked, or raw)
- **avocado** (all fresh, frozen, cooked, or raw)
- **bamboo shoots** (all fresh, frozen, cooked, or raw)
- **beets** (all fresh, frozen, cooked, or raw)
- **bitter melon** (all fresh, frozen, cooked, or raw)
- **Brussels sprouts** (all fresh, frozen, cooked, or raw)
- **green cabbage** (all fresh, frozen, cooked, or raw)
- **savoy cabbage** (all fresh, frozen, cooked, or raw)
- **red cabbage** (all fresh, frozen, cooked, or raw)
- **cactus pads** (all fresh, frozen, cooked, or raw)
- **cauliflower** (all fresh, frozen, cooked, or raw)
- **celery** (all fresh, frozen, cooked, or raw)
- **chayote (mirliton)** (all fresh, frozen, cooked, or raw)
- **cucumber** (all fresh, frozen, cooked, or raw)
- **eggplant** (all fresh, frozen, cooked, or raw)
- **green beans** (all fresh, frozen, cooked, or raw)
- **kohlrabi** (all fresh, frozen, cooked, or raw)
- **luffa** (all fresh, frozen, cooked, or raw)
- **mushrooms** (all fresh, frozen, cooked, or raw)
- **okra** (all fresh, frozen, cooked, or raw)
- **onions** (all fresh, frozen, cooked, or raw)

- **radish** (all fresh, frozen, cooked, or raw)
- **rutabaga** (all fresh, frozen, cooked, or raw)
- **seaweed** (all fresh, frozen, cooked, or raw)
- **snow peas** (all fresh, frozen, cooked, or raw)
- **summer squash** (all fresh, frozen, cooked, or raw)
- **tomatillos** (all fresh, frozen, cooked, or raw)

2. FRUITS

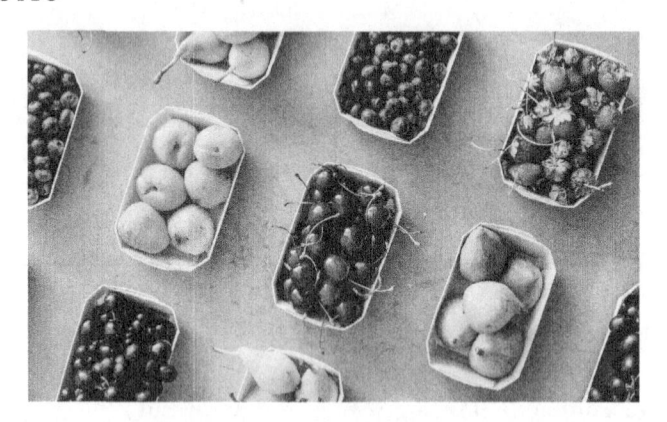

2.1 WHAT IS THE PORTION SIZE?

The typical serving sizes for fruits and fruits juices are equivalent to:

- 1 medium piece
- 1 cup (6 oz) of sliced fruits
- 3/4 cup (6 oz) of fruit juice

All fruits in this list are low-glycemic-index and anti-inflammatory

How Much a Day?

Up to 4 servings per day

THE ESSENTIAL FOODS LISTS FOR THE GLYCEMIC INDEX DIET

The fruit food group comprises whole fruits and fruit products (100% fruit juice). Whole fruits can be eaten in various forms, such as cut, cubed, sliced, or diced. At least 60% of the recommended amount of total fruit should come from whole fruit, rather than 100% juice. Juices should be without added sugars, food additives.

For most people, following the low-glycemic diet will require an increase in total fruit. Strategies to increase total fruit intake include

1. consuming often fruits and in a variety:
2. adding fruits to breakfast.
3. choosing more whole fruits as snacks
4. blending and consuming fruits into smoothies
5. choosing and carrying fruit with you to eat later
6. creating adequate pairings with your favorite foods

- **apples** (all fresh, frozen, dried fruits or 100% fruit juices)
- **Asian pears** (all fresh, frozen, dried fruits or 100% fruit juices)
- **bananas** (all fresh, frozen, dried fruits or 100% fruit juices)
- **blackberries** (all fresh, frozen, dried fruits or 100% fruit juices)
- **blueberries** (all fresh, frozen, dried fruits or 100% fruit juices)
- **currants** (all fresh, frozen, dried fruits or 100% fruit juices)
- **huckleberries** (all fresh, frozen, dried fruits or 100% fruit juices)
- **kiwifruit** (all fresh, frozen, dried fruits or 100% fruit juices)
- **mulberries** (all fresh, frozen, dried fruits or 100% fruit juices)
- **raspberries** (all fresh, frozen, dried fruits or 100% fruit juices)
- **strawberries** (all fresh, frozen, dried fruits or 100% fruit juices)

- **calamondin** (all fresh, frozen, dried fruits or 100% fruit juices)
- **grapefruit** (all fresh, frozen, dried fruits or 100% fruit juices)
- **lemons** (all fresh, frozen, dried fruits or 100% fruit juices)
- **limes** (all fresh, frozen, dried fruits or 100% fruit juices)
- **oranges** (all fresh, frozen, dried fruits or 100% fruit juices)
- **pomelos** (all fresh, frozen, dried fruits or 100% fruit juices)
- **cherries** (all fresh, frozen, dried fruits or 100% fruit juices)
- **dates** (all fresh, frozen, dried fruits or 100% fruit juices)
- **figs** (all fresh, frozen, dried fruits or 100% fruit juices)
- **grapes** (all fresh, frozen, dried fruits or 100% fruit juices)
- **guava** (all fresh, frozen, dried fruits or 100% fruit juices)
- **lychee** (all fresh, frozen, dried fruits or 100% fruit juices)
- **mangoes** (all fresh, frozen, dried fruits or 100% fruit juices)
- **nectarines** (all fresh, frozen, dried fruits or 100% fruit juices)
- **peaches** (all fresh, frozen, dried fruits or 100% fruit juices)
- **pears** (all fresh, frozen, dried fruits or 100% fruit juices)
- **plums** (all fresh, frozen, dried fruits or 100% fruit juices)
- **pomegranates** (all fresh, frozen, dried fruits or 100% fruit juices)
- **rhubarb** (all fresh, frozen, dried fruits or 100% fruit juices)
- **sapote** (all fresh, frozen, dried fruits or 100% fruit juices)
- **soursop** (all fresh, frozen, dried fruits or 100% fruit juices)

3. GRAINS

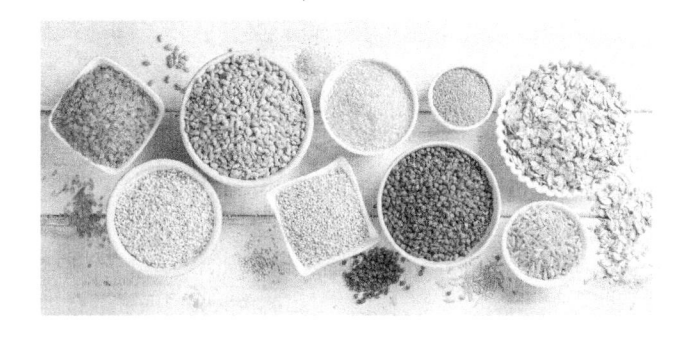

3.1 WHAT IS THE PORTION SIZE?

The typical serving sizes for cereals and grains are equivalent to:

- ⅓ cup breakfast cereal or muesli
- ½ cup of cooked cereal, or other cooked grain
- ⅓ cup of cooked rice (white rice excluded), and other small grains
- ½ cup of cold cereal

All breakfast cereal in this list are low-glycemic-index and anti-inflammatory

How Much a Day?

Up to 3 servings per day.

3.2 Whole grains

- **barley** (all whole-grain products or used as ingredients)
- **brown rice** (all whole-grain products or used as ingredients)
- **buckwheat** (all whole-grain products or used as ingredients)
- **bulgur** (all whole-grain products or used as ingredients)
- **millet** (all whole-grain products or used as ingredients)
- **oats (Avena sativa L.)** (all whole-grain products or used as ingredients)

- **quinoa** (all whole-grain products or used as ingredients)
- **dark rye** (all whole-grain products or used as ingredients)
- **whole-wheat bread** (all whole-grain products or used as ingredients)
- **whole-wheat chapati** (all whole-grain products or used as ingredients)
- **whole-grain cereals** (all whole-grain products or used as ingredients)
- **wild rice** (all whole-grain products or used as ingredients)

4. DAIRY AND FORTIFIED SOY ALTERNATIVES

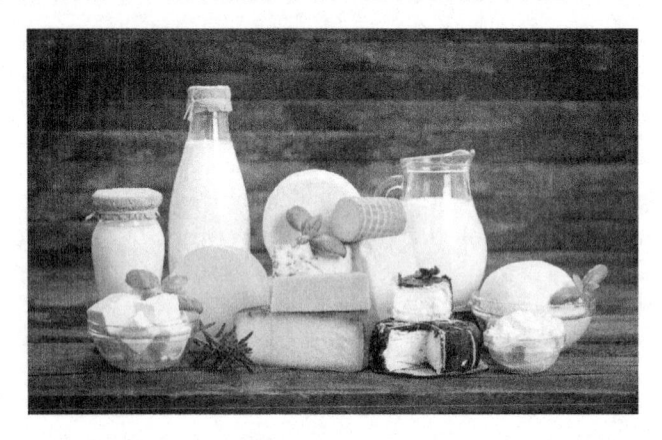

4.1 WHAT IS THE PORTION SIZE?

The typical serving sizes for dairy products are equivalent to:

- 1 cup of milk, soy beverage, or yogurt
- ⅓ cup of cottage cheese
- 1 oz of cheese

All dairy and soy alternatives in this list are low-glycemic-index and anti-inflammatory.

THE ESSENTIAL FOODS LISTS FOR THE GLYCEMIC INDEX DIET

People with celiac disease or lactose intolerance should consume dairy alternatives

How Much a Day?

Up to 3 servings per day

- **buttermilk** (all fluid, evaporated milk, or dry including lactose-free and lactose-reduced products)
- **soy beverages** (all fluid, evaporated milk, or dry including lactose-free and lactose-reduced products)
- **soy milk** (all fluid, evaporated milk, or dry including lactose-free and lactose-reduced products)
- **yogurt** (without added sugar and food additives) (all fluid, evaporated milk, or dry including lactose-free and lactose-reduced products)
- **kefir** (without added sugar and food additives) (all fluid, evaporated milk, or dry including lactose-free and lactose-reduced products)
- **frozen yogurt** (without added sugar and food additives) (all fluid, evaporated milk, or dry including lactose-free and lactose-reduced products)
- **cheeses** (all fluid, evaporated milk, or dry including lactose-free and lactose-reduced products)

---

5. PROTEIN FOODS

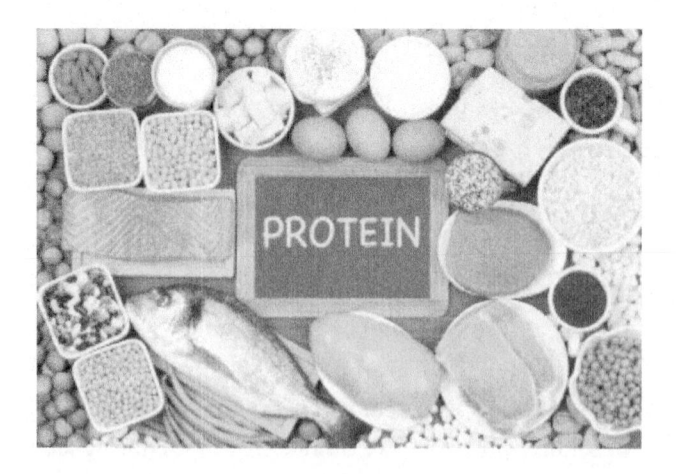

Eating an adequate amount of protein is extremely important for your health. Because Protein plays a crucial role in your body's vital processes and metabolisms, such as building and repairing tissues, building muscles, blood, hair, and skin, and producing hormones, enzymes, and other body chemicals.

Unlike carbohydrates and fat, your body does not store protein, and you need to eat the necessary amount to keep the right hormonal balance and fight unnecessary inflammation. Animal-based foods are identified as superior sources of protein because they offer a complete composition of essential amino acids, with higher bioavailability and digestibility (>90%). Therefore, the main principle to observe here when designing your meal program is to keep a weekly proteins intake equivalent to:

- 30 servings of animal proteins (mainly lean white meat and eggs)
- 10 servings of seafood
- 5 servings of nuts and seeds

THE ESSENTIAL FOODS LISTS FOR THE GLYCEMIC INDEX DIET

5.1 MEATS, POULTRY, EGGS, SEAFOODS: WHAT IS THE PORTION SIZE?

The typical serving sizes for the "meats, poultry, eggs", "seafood", and "nuts, seeds, soy Products" groups are equivalent to:

- 3 to 4 ounces of cooked, baked, or broiled beef
- 3 to 4 ounces of cooked, baked, or broiled veal
- 3 to 4 ounces of cooked, baked, or broiled poultry
- 3 to 4 ounces of cooked or canned fish
- 3 to 4 ounces of seafood
- 2 medium eggs
- ⅓ cup of nuts (5 large or 10 small nuts)
- 2 tablespoons of nut butter
- 2 tablespoons of nut spread

5.2 Meats, Poultry, Eggs

Meats (lean or low-fats) include:

- beef, goat, lamb, pork (fat red meats must be limited due to their pro-inflammatory effects). You have to choose lean meats preferably grass-fed beef, lamb, or bison
- game meat (e.g., bison, moose, elk, deer)

Poultry (lean or low-fats) includes

- chicken
- turkey
- cornish hens
- duck
- game birds (e.g., ostrich, pheasant, and quail)
- goose.

Eggs include

- chicken eggs
- turkey eggs
- duck eggs and other birds' eggs

5.3 Seafood

Seafood include

- salmon
- sardine
- anchovy
- black sea bass
- catfish
- clams
- cod
- crab
- crawfish
- flounder
- haddock
- hake
- herring
- lobster
- mullet
- oyster
- perch
- pollock
- scallop
- shrimp
- sole
- squid
- tilapia

- freshwater trout
- tuna

5.4 Nuts, Seeds, Soy Products

Nuts (and nut butter) include

- almonds
- pecans
- Brazil nuts
- pistachios
- hazelnuts
- macadamias
- pine nuts
- walnuts
- cashew nuts

Seeds (and seed butter) include:

- pumpkin seeds
- psyllium seeds
- chia seeds.
- flax seeds
- sunflower seeds
- sesame seeds
- poppy seeds

PART II
YOUR GROCERY SHOPPING LIST FOR LOW GI FOODS

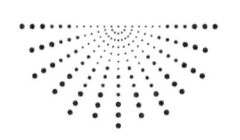

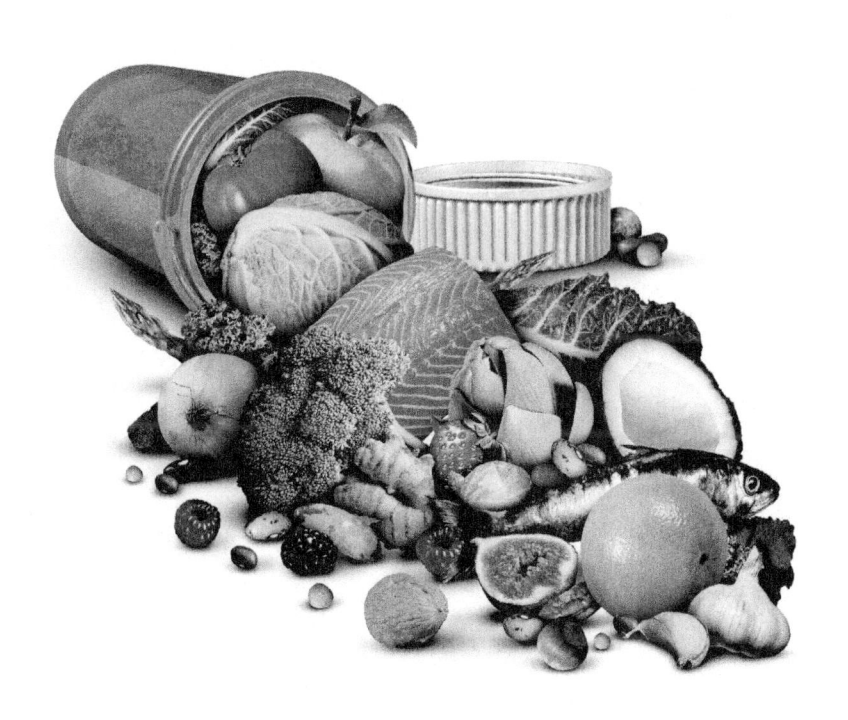

10
PORTIONS & SERVING SIZES

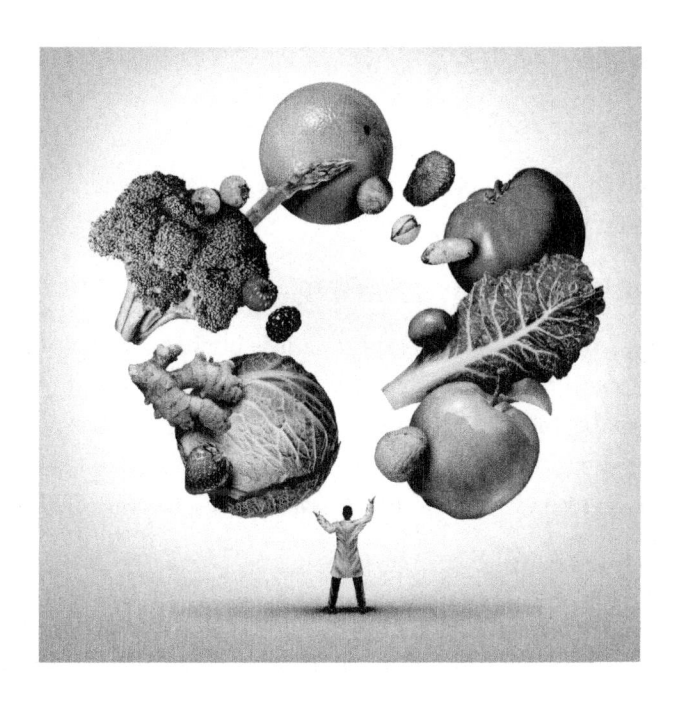

The twinkie diet explained

The twinkie diet refers to an experiment conducted a few years ago by Mark Haub, professor of nutrition at Kansas State University. He set out to discredit the claim of many diets' specialists, arguing that Calorie-counting is entirely irrelevant and unnecessary for weight loss. HAUB wasn't trying to claim that eating junk food (cream cakes, cookies, chips, snacks) is beneficial to your health, but he only demonstrates that if the Calories are deficient, weight loss is possible despite the quality of what a person eats.

Mark HAUB was limited to an intake of 1800 Calories a day while his daily requirements are about 2600 Calories, which made a daily caloric deficit of 800 Calories.

At the end of the experiment, he lost weight as he expected.

• His bodyweight went from 207 down to 174 pounds. His body mass index (BMI) dropped from 28.8 (overweight) to 24.9 (normal).

• His LDL (bad cholesterol) dropped by 20%

• His HDL (good cholesterol) increased by 20%

• His triglycerides (a type of fat (lipid) found in the blood) dropped by 39 per cent.

• His body fat went down from 33.4 to 24.9%

The main conclusion of the experiment is obvious: the caloric deficit works. However, you have to notice that calories are not equal. You have to make intelligent choices and choose high-quality food by following the guidelines in chapter 2, "Carbohydrates, Proteins and Fats: How macronutrient fit into a healthy low-glycemic diet?"

Portions sizes matter

Following the low-glycemic Index Diet looks simple because you need to know where different foods fall on the 0 to 100 glycemic index (GI).

• You fill up on low-glycemic index foods (GI value: 55 and under)

THE ESSENTIAL FOODS LISTS FOR THE GLYCEMIC INDEX DIET

• Eat smaller amounts of medium-glycemic index foods (GI value:56 to 69)

• And mostly avoid high-glycemic-index foods (GI value: 70 and up)

For weight loss, you have to pay closer attention to the portions sizes. After all, you may never lose weight despite choosing mainly low-glycemic foods and balancing them with medium-glycemic and high-glycemic foods. Recall the Mark Haub because you may never reach the calorie deficit needed to lose weight.

The glycemic load may be an essential tool to keep your total daily calories low, so use the GL to control your portion when possible.

Otherwise, you have also to use the serving sizes given below to identify the appropriate portion sizes of different foods for calorie control. Use the following recommendations as a general reference to determine the appropriate portion size.

ESTIMATE PORTION SIZES USING YOUR HAND

PORTION SIZE

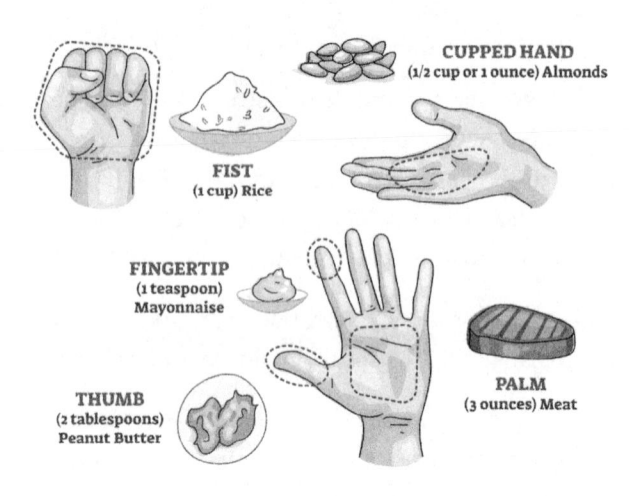

FIST
(1 cup) Rice

CUPPED HAND
(1/2 cup or 1 ounce) Almonds

FINGERTIP
(1 teaspoon) Mayonnaise

THUMB
(2 tablespoons) Peanut Butter

PALM
(3 ounces) Meat

This portion size measuring guide will help you estimate the amount of food on the plate without having to measure your portions.

The Palm

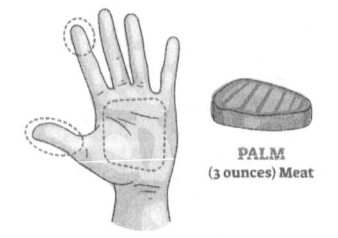

PALM
(3 ounces) Meat

The palm of your hand as shown in this figure may be used to estimate your protein intake. 1 palm is equivalent to a 3 ounces (oz.) serving of protein.

Examples of what you could estimate a 3-ounce serving include poultry, beef, fish, pork, and chicken.

The fist

A fist-sized portion is a great way of estimating a portion size of carbohydrates. You can use your fist to measure your intake of vegetables, fruits, cereals, and grains. 1 fist is equivalent to 1 cup.

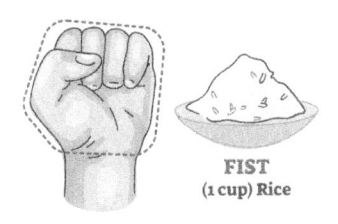

THE ESSENTIAL FOODS LISTS FOR THE GLYCEMIC INDEX DIET

FIST
(1 cup) Rice

. . .

Tip of Thumb

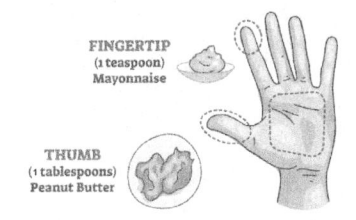

FINGERTIP
(1 teaspoon)
Mayonnaise

THUMB
(1 tablespoons)
Peanut Butter

The tip of a thumb is a great tool to estimate a portion size of healthy fat. You can use your tip of the thumb to estimate your fat intakes such as peanut butter, cheese, homemade salad dressings, butter. 1 thumb is equivalent to 1 tablespoon.

The fingertip

The fingertip is used to estimate the amount of healthy oils or fats you would consume. You can use your fingertip to measure your fat intakes such as nut butter, olive oil, homemade salad dressings, butter. 1 fingertip is equivalent to 1 teaspoon.

A Cupped Hand

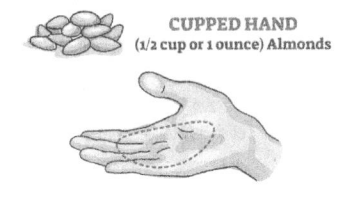

CUPPED HAND
(1/2 cup or 1 ounce) Almonds

The cupped hand is used to measure the amount of some foods such as nuts and seeds you would consume. You can use the surface area of your cupped hand to estimate a portion of seeds and nuts for example. 1 hand cupped is equivalent to a 1/2 cup.

Portions Sizes

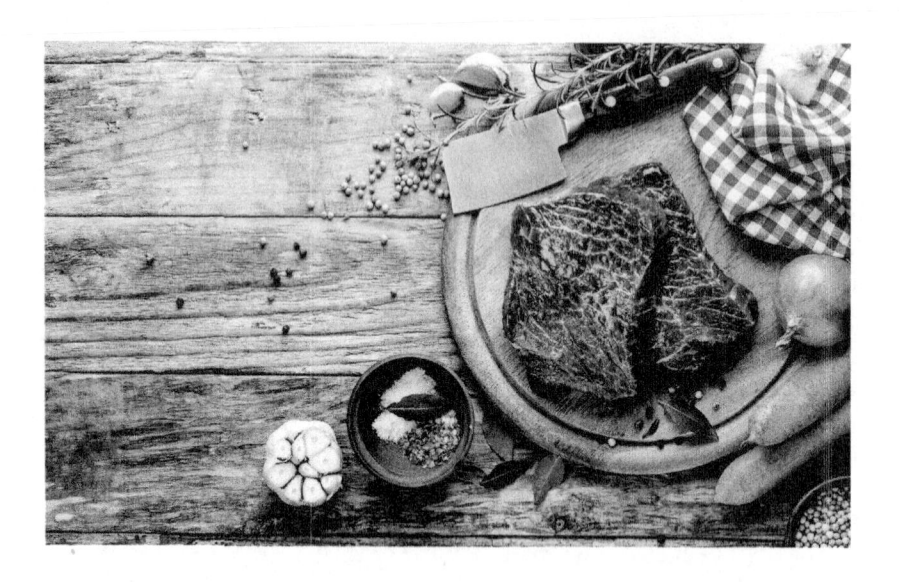

BEEF, LAMP, VEAL, PORK & POULTRY: WHAT IS THE PORTION SIZE?

The typical serving size for low GI Meats is equivalent to:

- 3 to 4 ounces of cooked, baked, broiled, or canned beef
- 3 to 4 ounces of cooked, baked, broiled, or canned veal
- 3 to 4 ounces of cooked, baked, broiled, or canned poultry
- 3 to 4 ounces of cooked, baked, broiled, or canned fork
- 2 medium eggs

For moderate GI Beef, Lamb, Veal, Pork & Poultry products reduce the serving by 1/3

How Much a Day?

THE ESSENTIAL FOODS LISTS FOR THE GLYCEMIC INDEX DIET

Up to 3 servings per day

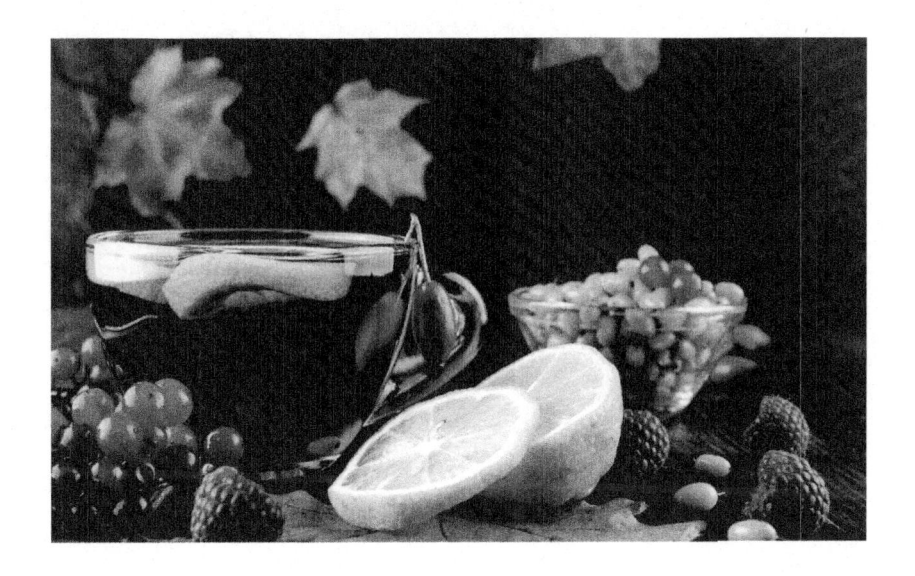

BEVERAGES: WHAT IS THE PORTION SIZE?

The typical serving size for low GI beverages is equivalent to:

- 1 cup (8 ounces) 100% vegetable juice
- ¾ cup (6 ounces) 100% fruit juice
- ¾ cup of soft drink
- 1 cup of (8 ounces) milk or yogurt drink

For moderate GI beverages products reduce the serving by 1/3

How Much a Day?

Up to 3 servings per day provided you respect your calorie deficit in your overall daily intake.

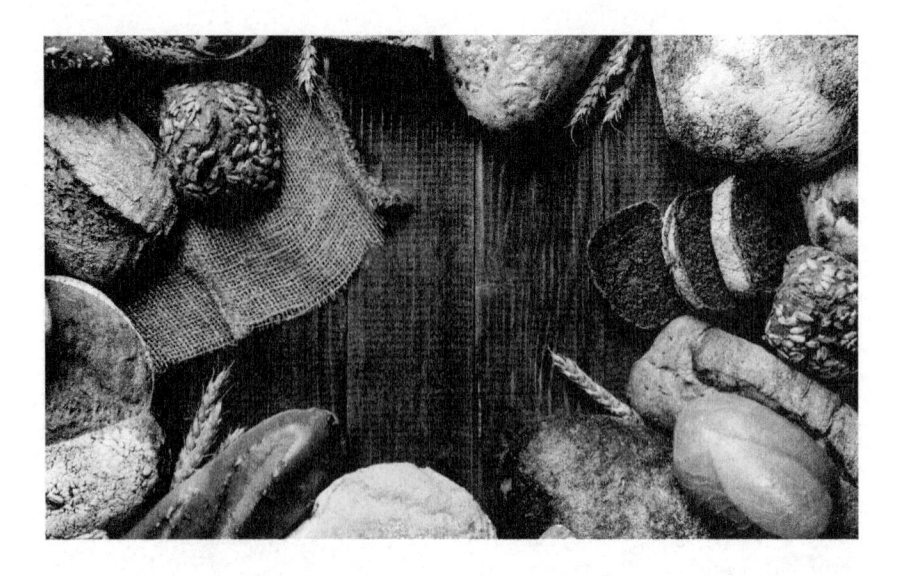

BREADS & BAKERY PRODUCTS: WHAT IS THE SERVING SIZE?

The typical serving size for low GI bread and bakery products is equivalent to:

- 1 slice bread
- ½ of muffin, bagel, or hamburger bun
- ½ slice of bakery products
- ½ cup cereal

For moderate GI bread and bakery products reduce the serving by 1/3

How Much a Day?

Up to 8 servings per day

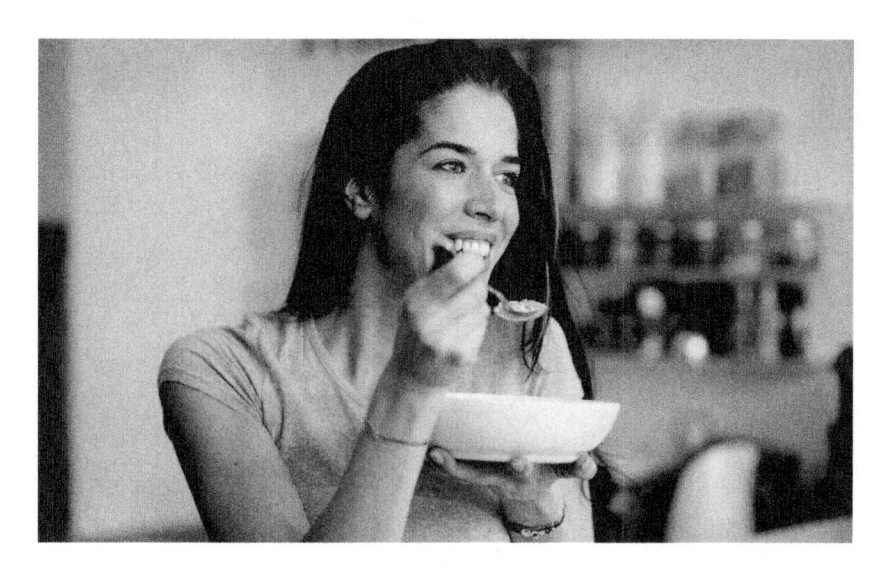

THE ESSENTIAL FOODS LISTS FOR THE GLYCEMIC INDEX DIET

GRAINS & BREAKFAST CEREALS: WHAT IS THE PORTION SIZE?

The typical serving sizes for low GI Breakfast Cereals are equivalent to:

- ⅓ cup breakfast cereal or muesli
- ½ cup of cooked cereal, pasta, or other cooked grain
- ⅓ cup of cooked rice, and other small grains
- ¾ cup of cold cereal

For moderate GI Grains & Breakfast Cereals reduce the serving by 1/3

How Much a Day?

Up to 8 servings per day provided you respect your calorie deficit in your overall daily intake.

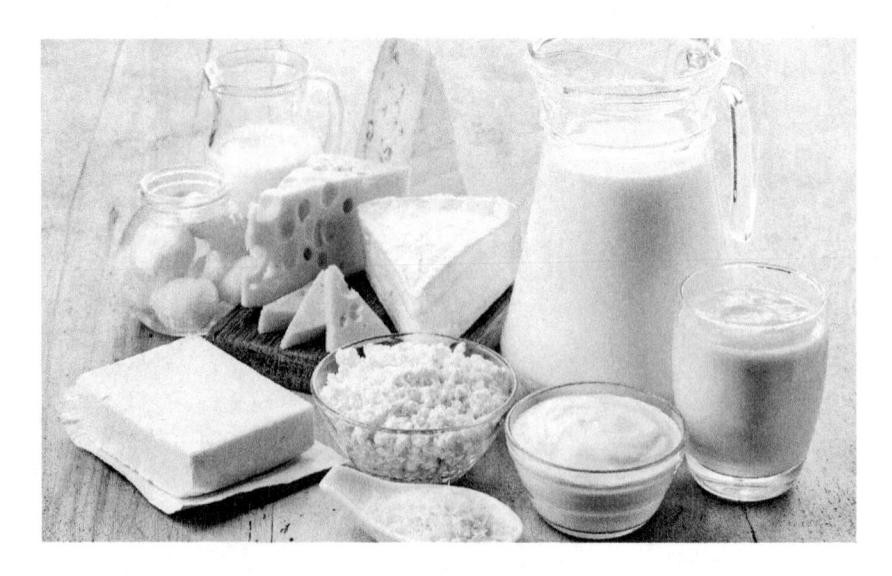

DAIRY PRODUCTS & ALTERNATIVES: WHAT IS THE PORTION SIZE?

The typical serving size for low GI dairy products & oils is equivalent to:

- 1 cup of milk or yogurt
- ⅓ cup of cottage cheese
- 1 oz of cheese
- 1 teaspoon of oil or butter
- 1 teaspoon of margarine, or mayonnaise

For moderate GI Dairy Products & Alternatives reduce the serving by 1/3

How Much a Day?

Up to 3 servings per day

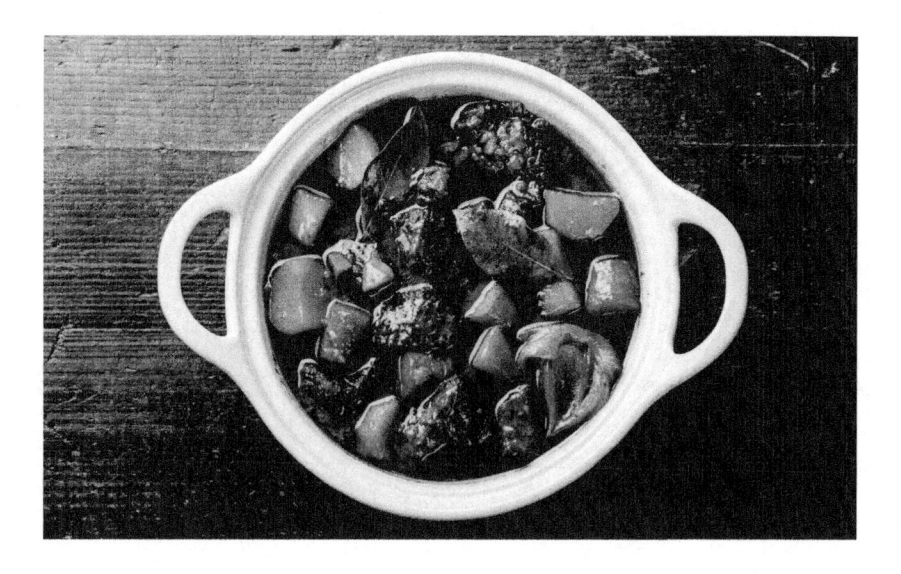

SOUPS, PASTA AND NOODLES: WHAT IS THE PORTION SIZE?

The typical serving sizes for low GI Soups, Pasta, and Noodles are equivalent to:

- 1 cup vegetable soup
- ½ cup of cooked cereal, pasta, or other cooked grain
- ⅓ cup of cooked rice, and other small grains

For moderate GI Soups, Pasta and Noodles reduce the serving by 1/3

How Much a Day?

Up to 8 servings per day provided you respect your calorie deficit in your overall daily intake.

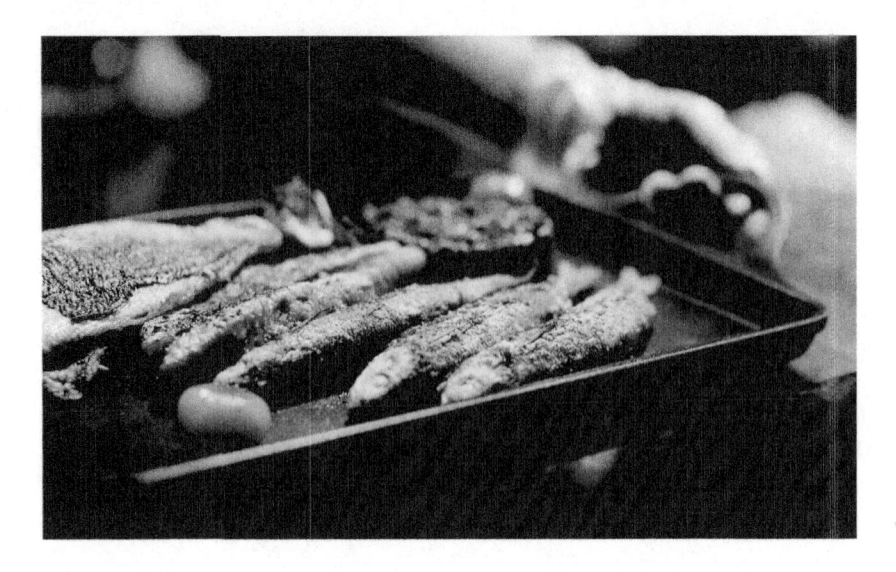

FISH & FISH PRODUCTS: WHAT IS THE PORTION SIZE?

The typical serving sizes for low GI Fishes & Fishes Products are equivalent to:

- 3 to 4 ounces of cooked or canned fish
- 3 to 4 ounces of seafood

For moderate GI Fish & Fish Products reduce the serving by 1/3

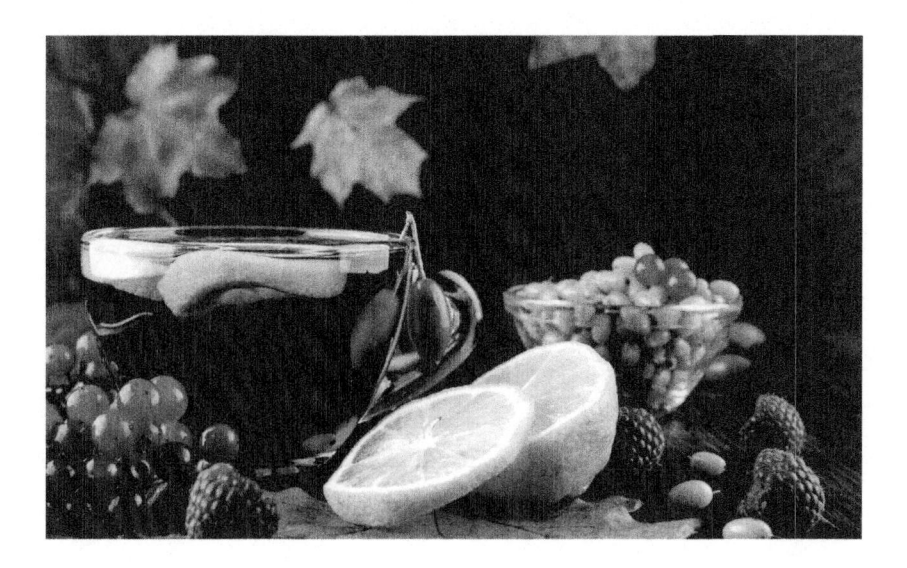

THE ESSENTIAL FOODS LISTS FOR THE GLYCEMIC INDEX DIET

FRUIT AND FRUIT PRODUCTS: WHAT IS THE PORTION SIZE?

The typical serving sizes for low GI fruits and fruits juices are equivalent to:

- 1 medium piece of low GI or moderate GI fruit
- 1 cup of canned or sliced fruits
- 3/4 cup (6 oz) of fruit juice

For moderate GI fruits and fruits juices reduce the serving by 1/3

How Much a Day?

Up to 4 servings per day

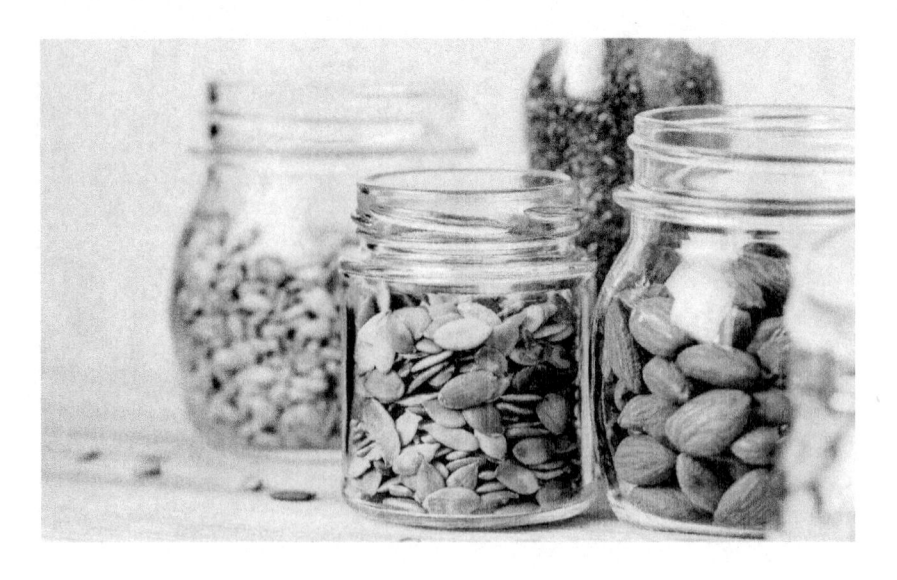

LEGUMES AND NUTS: WHAT IS THE PORTION SIZE?

The typical serving sizes for low GI legumes and nuts are equivalent to:

- ⅓ cup of nuts (5 large or 10 small nuts)
- ½ cup of cooked or canned beans, lentils, and chickpeas
- 2 tablespoons of nut butter
- 2 tablespoons of nut spread

For moderate GI Legumes and Nuts reduce the serving by 1/3

How Much a Day?

Up to 3 servings per day (because nuts and beans are generally dense in calories)

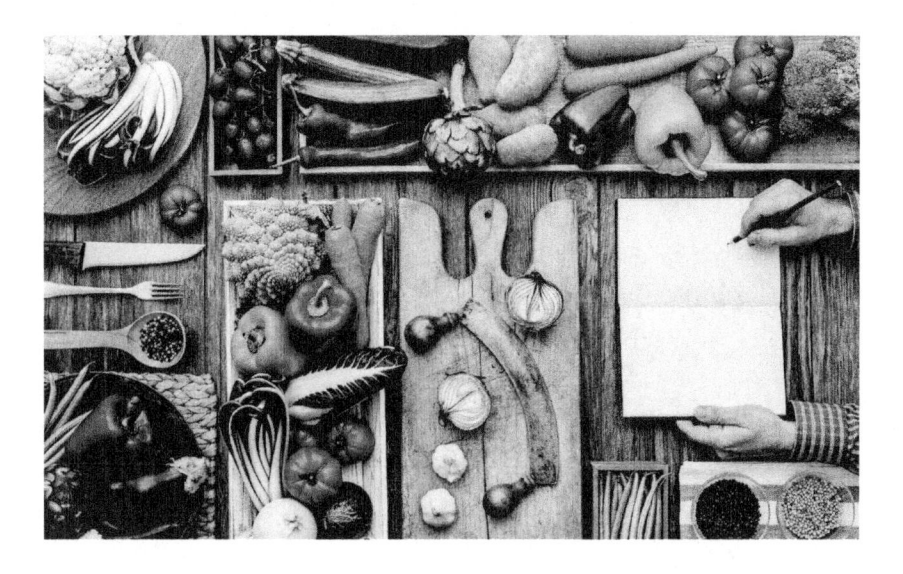

VEGETABLES: WHAT IS THE PORTION SIZE?

The typical serving sizes for low GI vegetables and vegetable juices can be expressed as

- 1 cup raw or salad vegetables
- 1/2 cup cooked or canned vegetables
- 3/4 cup (6oz) vegetable juice homemade and unsweetened

For moderate GI vegetables and vegetable juices reduce the serving by 1/3

How Much a Day?

Up to 10 servings per day

11

BEVERAGES: LOW AND MEDIUM GLYCEMIC INDEX FOODS

The 2020-2025 Dietary Guidelines for Americans advises that adults of legal drinking age may choose not to drink at all or to drink in moderation by restricting intake to a maximum of 2 drinks for men or 1 drink or less for women in a day—on days when alcohol is consumed.

- Alcoholic Beverage—100 Proof ⟶ 0.0 (Low)
- Alcoholic Beverage—86 Proof ⟶ 0.0 (Low)
- Alcoholic Beverage—90 Proof ⟶ 0.0 (Low)
- Alcoholic Beverage—94 Proof ⟶ 0.0 (Low)
- Alcoholic Beverage—Amber Hard Cider ⟶ 38-44 (Low)
- Alcoholic Beverage—Black Russian ⟶ 0.0 (Low)
- Alcoholic Beverage—Bloody Mary ⟶ 31-35 (Low)
- Alcoholic Beverage—Brandy ⟶ 0.0 (Low)

THE ESSENTIAL FOODS LISTS FOR THE GLYCEMIC INDEX DIET

- Alcoholic Beverage—Cabernet Franc ► 0 (Low)
- Alcoholic Beverage—Cabernet Sauvignon ► 0 (Low)
- Alcoholic Beverage—Champagne Punch ► 0 (Low)
- Alcoholic Beverage—Chardonnay ► 0 (Low)
- Alcoholic Beverage—Chenin Blanc ► 0 (Low)
- Alcoholic Beverage—Gin ► 0.0 (Low)
- Alcoholic Beverage—Pina Colada ► 15 (Low)
- Alcoholic Beverage—Pina Colada Homemade ► 15 (Low)
- Alcoholic Beverage—Root Beer, sugar free ► 0 (Low)
- Alcoholic Beverage—Rum ► 0.0 (Low)
- Alcoholic Beverage—Sake ► 66 (Medium)
- Alcoholic Beverage—Sangria ► 50 (Low)
- Alcoholic Beverage—Tequila ► 0.0 (Low)
- Alcoholic Beverage—Vodka ► 0.0 (Low)
- Alcoholic Beverage—Whiskey ► 0.0 (Low)
- Alcoholic Beverage—Whiskey Sour ► 50 (Low)
- Alcoholic Beverage—Whiskey Sour Canned ► 50 (Low)
- Alcoholic Beverage—Wine, red ► 0.0 (Low)
- Alcoholic Beverage—Wine, white ► 0.0 (Low)
- Apple cider ► 40 (Low)
- Cacao powder ► 24 (Low)
- Carob powder ► 41 (Low)
- Chicory Beverage ► 40 (Low)

- Chicory coffee ➜ 0.0 (Low)
- Chocolate syrup ➜ 55-68 (Medium)
- Chocolate—Ice cream soda ➜ 59.5 (Medium)
- Coca Cola ➜ 63 (Medium)
- Coca Cola ➜ 63 (Medium)
- Cocoa drink— low-fat milk added ➜ 37.5 (Low)
- Cocoa drink— milk added ➜ 37 (Low)
- Cocoa drink—dry milk, water added ➜ 37.5 (Low)
- Cocoa drink—hot chocolate, whole milk ➜ 36 (Low)
- Cocoa drink—nonfat milk and low-calorie sweetener ➜ 24 (Low)
- Cocoa drink—skim milk added ➜ 37.5 (Low)
- Cocoa Drink—whey, low-fat milk added ➜ 24 (Low)
- Cocoa drink—whole milk added ➜ 36 (Low)
- Cocoa powder ➜ 24 (Low)
- Coconut water—fresh ➜ 41 (Low)
- Coconut water—packaged ➜ 54 (Low)
- Coffee—Bottled or canned ➜ 50 (Low)
- Coffee—Brewed ➜ 50 (Low)
- Coffee—Brewed Blend Of Decaffeinated ➜ 50 (Low)
- Coffee—Brewed Blend Of Regular ➜ 50 (Low)
- Coffee—Brewed Espresso Decaffeinated ➜ 50 (Low)
- Coffee—Cafe Con Leche ➜ 58 (Medium)
- Coffee—Cafe Con Leche Decaffeinated ➜ 58 (Medium)

THE ESSENTIAL FOODS LISTS FOR THE GLYCEMIC INDEX DIET

- Coffee—Café Latte (soy milk) ➧ 37 (Low)
- Coffee—Cafe Mocha ➧ 58-68 (Medium)
- Coffee—Cafe Mocha Decaffeinated ➧ 58-68 (Medium)
- Coffee—Cafe Mocha Decaffeinated ➧ 58-68 (Medium)
- Coffee—decaffeinated, made from powdered instant ➧ 50 (Low)
- Coffee—espresso ➧ 50 (Low)
- Coffee—espresso, decaffeinated ➧ 50 (Low)
- Coffee—from ground ➧ 50 (Low)
- Coffee—from ground decaffeinated ➧ 50 (Low)
- Coffee—from ground, 50% regular and 50% decaffeinated ➧ 50 (Low)
- Coffee—from ground, regular ➧ 50 (Low)
- Coffee—from liquid concentrate ➧ 50 (Low)
- Coffee—from powdered instant mix with sugar ➧ 68 (Low)
- Coffee—from powdered instant mix, low-calorie sweetener ➧ 27 (Low)
- Coffee—from powdered instant mix, with whitener and sugar, instant ➧ 47.5 (Low)
- Coffee—instant decaffeinated, and chicory ➧ 50 (Low)
- Coffee—latte ➧ 68 (Medium)
- Coffee—presweetened with sugar ➧ 66.4 (Medium)
- Coffee—rom ground, flavored ➧ 50 (Low)
- Cream soda ➧ 55-68 (Medium)
- Creamer powder ➧ 16-30 (Low)

- Diet beverage ☞ 30-54 (Low)
- Diet Coke ☞ 0 (Low)
- Diet Cola ☞ 0 (Low)
- Diet Green Tea ☞ 0 (Low)
- Diet Pepper Cola ☞ 0 (Low)
- Drink—Acai Berry Fortified ☞ 24.2 (Low)
- Drink—Acai Berry Unsweetned ☞ 24.2 (Low)
- Drink—Apricot orange vitamin C added ☞ 47-51 (Low)
- Drink—Carbonated citrus ☞ 61-65 (Medium)
- Drink—Chocolate-flavored Beverage unsweetened ☞ 50 (Low)
- Drink—Cranberry apple juice ☞ 52 (Low)
- Drink—Cranberry apple juice low-calorie ☞ 48 (Low)
- Drink—Cranberry apple juice vitamin C added ☞ 52 (Low)
- Drink—Cranberry juice ☞ 58-61 (Medium)
- Drink—Cranberry juice low-calorie ☞ 47-51 (Low)
- Drink—Cranberry juice with vitamin C added ☞ 58-61 (Medium)
- Drink—Fruit-flavored thirst quencher beverage, low-calorie ☞ 50 (Low)
- Drink—Fruit-flavored, from low-calorie powdered mix ☞ 50 (Low)
- Drink—Fruit-flavored, from powdered mix ☞ 68 (Medium)
- Drink—Fruit-flavored, from sweetened powdered mix ☞ 68 (Medium)
- Drink—Fruit-flavored, punches, ades, low-calorie ☞ 50 (Low)

- Drink—Grapefruit juice, low-calorie ► 50 (Low)
- Drink—Grapefruit juice, vitamin C added, low-calorie ► 50 (Low)
- Drink—Grapefruit Orange juice ► 48 (Low)
- Drink—Grapefruit Orange juice low-calorie ► 47 (Low)
- Drink—Milk with chocolate (average) ► 37 (Low)
- Drink—Milk with chocolate made with skim milk (average) ► 37.5 (Low)
- Drink—Milk with chocolate made with whole milk (average) ► 36 (Low)
- Drink—Milk with chocolate, low-fat (average) ► 37.5 (Low)
- Drink—Orange breakfast ► 68 (Medium)
- Drink—Orange breakfast from frozen ► 68 (Medium)
- Drink—Orange breakfast Low-calorie ► 50 (Low)
- Drink—Orange Cranberry Juice ► 49-54 (Low)
- Drink—Whey and milk-beverage, Chocolate-flavored ► 37.5 (Low)
- Espresso—decaffeinated ► 0.0 (Low)
- Espresso—regular ► 0.0 (Low)
- Fanta ► 68 (Medium)
- Ginger beer, sugar-free ► 0.0 (Low)
- Grape juice, unsweetened ► 45 (Low)
- Ice cream soda ► 64.5 (Medium)
- Juice—Aloe Vera ► 58-69 (Medium)
- Juice—Aloe Vera Vitamin C Fortified ► 58-69 (Medium)

- Juice—Apple & Raspberry from fresh ☞ 40 (Low)
- Juice—Apple cherry ☞ 40-44 (Low)
- Juice—Apple cherry ☞ 41-45 (Low)
- Juice—Apple grape ☞ 40-44 (Low)
- Juice—Apple pear ☞ 40-44 (Low)
- Juice—Apple raspberry ☞ 40-44 (Low)
- Juice—Apple raspberry grape ☞ 40-44 (Low)
- Juice—Apple, 99% —from fresh ☞ 41 (Low)
- Juice—Apple, 99% —reconstituted ☞ 50 (Low)
- Juice—Apricot ☞ 54 (Low)
- Juice—Apricot orange ☞ 47-51 (Low)
- Juice—Banana ☞ 58-69 (Medium)
- Juice—Carbonated citrus, low-calorie ☞ 49-52 (Low)
- Juice—Celery ☞ 32 (Low)
- Juice—Cherry ☞ 22-28 (Low)
- Juice—Cherry Canned ☞ 22-28 (Low)
- Juice—Cranberry apple ☞ 48 (Low)
- Juice—Cranberry red grape, unsweetened ☞ 66-69 (Medium)
- Juice—Cranberry white grape, unsweetened ☞ 66-69 (Medium)
- Juice—Cranberry, unsweetened ☞ 68 (Medium)
- Juice—Fruit cocktail ☞ 55 (Low)
- Juice—Grape lemon tangerine ☞ 50 (Low)
- Juice—Grapefruit and orange ☞ 49 (Low)

THE ESSENTIAL FOODS LISTS FOR THE GLYCEMIC INDEX DIET

- Juice—Grapefruit and orange, unsweetened ☛ 49 (Low)

- Juice—Grapefruit unsweetened ☛ 48 (Low)

- Juice—Orange 25-50% from fresh ☛ 50 (Low)

- Juice—Orange and banana ☛ 50 (Low)

- Juice—Orange from fresh sweetened with sugar ☛ 60-69 (Medium)

- Juice—Orange from fresh unsweetened ☛ 50 (Low)

- Juice—Orange from frozen unsweetened ☛ 50 (Low)

- Juice—Orange from frozen, with calcium unsweetened ☛ 50 (Low)

- Juice—Orange from frozen, with vitamin D unsweetened ☛ 50 (Low)

- Juice—Orange juice fresh ☛ 50 (Low)

- Juice—Orange peach white grape ☛ 50-54 (Low)

- Juice—Orange unsweetened ☛ 50 (Low)

- Juice—Orange, 98% reconstituted ☛ 50 (Low)

- Juice—Orange, 99% reconstituted ☛ 50 (Low)

- Juice—Peach ☛ 38 (Low)

- Juice—Peach white grape orange ☛ 50 (Low)

- Juice—Pear ☛ 44 (Low)

- Juice—Pineapple apple guava ☛ 43 (Low)

- Juice—Pineapple apple guava with vitamin C ☛ 43 (Low)

- Juice—Pineapple grapefruit, unsweetened ☛ 47 (Low)

- Juice—Pineapple orange banana, unsweetened ☛ 48 (Low)

- Juice—Pineapple orange, unsweetened ► 48 (Low)
- Juice—Pineapple unsweetened ► 46 (Low)
- Juice—Pineapple with sugar ► 60-69 (Medium)
- Juice—Pineapple with vitamin C, unsweetened ► 46 (Low)
- Juice—Prune, unsweetened ► 45 (Low)
- Juice—Strawberry orange banana, unsweetened ► 50 (Low)
- Juice—Tomato ► 35 (Low)
- Juice—Tomato and vegetable ► 35-38 (Low)
- Lactose-free milk drink ► 15-30 (Low)
- Lemonade ► 54 (Low)
- Lemonade, low-calorie ► 16-30 (Low)
- Milkshake with malt ► 53 (Low)
- Milkshake—chocolate, made with skim milk ► 46.5 (Low)
- Milkshake—flavor or type (average) ► 44 (Low)
- Milkshake—flavors other than chocolate, made with skim milk ► 46.5 (Low)
- Milkshake—homemade, chocolate ► 44 (Low)
- Milkshake—homemade, flavors other than chocolate ► 44 (Low)
- Nonalcoholic malt beverage ► 40 (Low)
- Orange juice, No added Sugar (reconstituted) ► 50 (Low)
- Protein supplement, plant-based ► 28-44 (Low)
- Soft drink— sugar-free ► 50 (Low)
- Soft drink—average ► 63-69 (Medium)
- Soft drink—cola-type ► 63-69 (Medium)

THE ESSENTIAL FOODS LISTS FOR THE GLYCEMIC INDEX DIET

- Soft drink—cola-type, decaffeinated ← 63-69 (Medium)
- Soft drink—cola-type, high amount of caffeine ← 63-69 (Medium)
- Soft drink—cola-type, sugar-free, decaffeinated ← 50 (Low)
- Soft drink—cola-type, sugar-free ← 50 (Low)
- Soft drink—fruit-flavored with caffeine ← 63-69 (Medium)
- Soft drink—fruit-flavored, sugar-free, with caffeine ← 50 (Low)
- Soft drink—fruit-flavored ← 63-69 (Medium)
- Soft drink—pepper-type, sugar-free ← 50 (Low)
- Soft drink—pepper-type, sugar-free and decaffeinated, ← 50 (Low)
- Soft drink—sugar-free, fruit-flavored ← 50 (Low)
- Soft drink, cola-type ← 58-69 (Medium)
- Tea black—leaf, unsweetened ← Low
- Tea herbal—from chicory roots, ginger ← Low
- Tea herbal—from dried mint, lemon, and ginger ← Low
- Tea herbal—from fresh mint, lemon, and ginger ← Low
- Tea with fennel—made up with water ← Low
- Tea with licorice—made up with water ← Low
- Tea—Black Brewed ← 0 (Low)
- Tea—Black Ready to drink ← 0 (Low)
- Tea—chamomile ← 0 (Low)
- Tea—green, leaf, unsweetened ← 0 (Low)
- Water—Bottled ← 0 (Low)

12
BREADS: LOW AND MEDIUM GLYCEMIC INDEX FOODS

- Bagel—multigrain — 43 (Low)
- Bagel—multigrain, toasted — 43 (Low)
- Bagel—multigrain, with raisins — 43 (Low)
- Bagel—multigrain, with raisins, toasted — 43 (Low)
- Bagel—oat bran — 47 (Low)
- Bagel—oat bran, toasted — 47 (Low)
- Bagel—pumpernickel — 50 (Low)
- Bagel—pumpernickel, toasted — 50 (Low)
- Baklava — 59 (Medium)
- Bread—100% Whole Grain — 51 (Low)
- Bread—barley — 67 (Medium)
- Bread—dough, fried — 66 (Medium)
- Bread—fruit and nut — 57.9 (Medium)

- Bread—fruit, without nuts ☞ 57.9 (Medium)
- Bread—marble rye and pumpernickel ☞ 50 (Low)
- Bread—marble rye and pumpernickel, toasted ☞ 50 (Low)
- Bread—multigrain ☞ 43 (Low)
- Bread—multigrain, reduced-calorie and/or high fiber ☞ 43 (Low)
- Bread—multigrain, reduced-calorie and/or high fiber, toasted ☞ 43 (Low)
- Bread—multigrain, toasted ☞ 43 (Low)
- Bread—multigrain, with raisins ☞ 43 (Low)
- Bread—multigrain, with raisins, toasted ☞ 43 (Low)
- Bread—nut ☞ 57.9 (Medium)
- Bread—oat bran ☞ 31 (Low)
- Bread—oat bran, reduced-calorie and/or high fiber ☞ 31 (Low)
- Bread—oat bran, reduced-calorie and/or high fiber, toasted ☞ 31 (Low)
- Bread—oat bran, toasted ☞ 31 (Low)
- Bread—oatmeal ☞ 55 (Low)
- Bread—oatmeal, toasted ☞ 55 (Low)
- Bread—pita ☞ 57 (Medium)
- Bread—pita, toasted ☞ 57 (Medium)
- Bread—pita, wheat or cracked wheat ☞ 53 (Low)
- Bread—pita, wheat or cracked wheat, toasted ☞ 53 (Low)
- Bread—pumpernickel ☞ 50 (Low)
- Bread—pumpernickel, toasted ☞ 50 (Low)

- Bread—pumpkin ☞ 57.9 (Medium)
- Bread—raisin ☞ 63 (Medium)
- Bread—raisin, toasted ☞ 63 (Medium)
- Bread—reduced-calorie and/or high fiber, Italian ☞ 68 (Medium)
- Bread—reduced-calorie and/or high fiber, Italian, toasted ☞ 68 (Medium)
- Bread—reduced-calorie and/or high fiber, white ☞ 68 (Medium)
- Bread—reduced-calorie, white, toasted and/or high fiber, ☞ 68 (Medium)
- Bread—white, reduced-calorie with fruit and/or nuts, and/or high fiber ☞ 68 (Medium)
- Bread—reduced-calorie and/or high fiber, white, with fruit and/or nuts, toasted ☞ 68 (Medium)
- Bread—rice, toasted ☞ 66.5 (Medium)
- Bread—rye ☞ 58 (Medium)
- Bread—rye, reduced-calorie and/or high fiber ☞ 68 (Medium)
- Bread—rye, reduced-calorie and/or high fiber, toasted ☞ 68 (Medium)
- Bread—rye, toasted ☞ 58 (Medium)
- Bread—sourdough ☞ 54 (Low)
- Bread—sourdough, toasted ☞ 54 (Low)
- Bread—sprouted wheat, toasted ☞ 53 (Low)
- Bread—sunflower meal ☞ 57 (Medium)
- Bread—wheat or cracked wheat, made from home recipe or purchased at bakery ☞ 53 (Low)

- Bread—wheat or cracked wheat, made from home recipe or purchased at bakery, toasted ☛ 53 (Low)
- Bread—wheat or cracked wheat, with raisins ☛ 53 (Low)
- Bread—wheat or cracked wheat, with raisins, toasted ☛ 53 (Low)
- Bread—white, special formula, added fiber ☛ 68 (Medium)
- Bread—zucchini ☛ 57.9 (Medium)
- Cake—prepared with glutinous rice ☛ 64 (Medium)
- Cake—angel food, NS as to icing ☛ 67 (Medium)
- Cake—angel food, with fruit and icing or filling ☛ 67 (Medium)
- Cake—angel food, with icing ☛ 67 (Medium)
- Cake—angel food, without icing ☛ 67 (Medium)
- Cake—applesauce, NS as to icing ☛ 44 (Low)
- Cake—applesauce, with icing ☛ 44 (Low)
- Cake—applesauce, without icing ☛ 44 (Low)
- Cake—banana, NS as to icing ☛ 47 (Low)
- Cake—banana, with icing ☛ 47 (Low)
- Cake—banana, without icing ☛ 47 (Low)
- Cake—black forest made with chocolate and cherry ☛ 38 (Low)
- Cake—butter, with icing ☛ 42 (Low)
- Cake—butter, without icing ☛ 42 (Low)
- Cake—carrot, average for icing ☛ 62 (Medium)
- Cake—carrot, with icing ☛ 62 (Medium)
- Cake—carrot, without icing ☛ 62 (Medium)
- Cake—chocolate, made from home recipe, average for icing ☛

38 (Low)

🌿 Cake—chocolate, pudding type mix with light icing, light coating or light filling ☛ 38 (Low)

🌿 Cake—chocolate, pudding-type mix (oil, eggs, and water added to dry mix), icing not specified ☛ 38 (Low)

🌿 Cake—chocolate, pudding-type mix, with icing, filling or coating ☛ 38 (Low)

🌿 Cake—chocolate, pudding-type mix, without icing or filling ☛ 38 (Low)

🌿 Cake—chocolate, pudding-type mix, made by "Lite" recipe with filling, icing, or coating ☛ 38 (Low)

🌿 Cake—chocolate, standard-type mix, with filling, icing, or coating ☛ 38 (Low)

🌿 Cake—chocolate, standard-type mix, without icing or filling ☛ 38 (Low)

🌿 Cake—chocolate, with icing, coating, or filling, prepared from home recipe ☛ 38 (Low)

🌿 Cake—chocolate, with icing, coating, or filling, purchased ready-to-eat ☛ 38 (Low)

🌿 Cake—chocolate, without icing or filling, prepared from home recipe ☛ 38 (Low)

🌿 Cake—chocolate, without icing or filling, purchased ready-to-eat ☛ 38 (Low)

🌿 Cake—chocolate, with icing, light ☛ 38 (Low)

🌿 Cake—coconut, with icing ☛ 42 (Low)

🌿 Cake—cupCake, chocolate, icing not specified ☛ 38 (Low)

🌿 Cake—cupCake, chocolate, with icing or filling ☛ 38 (Low)

THE ESSENTIAL FOODS LISTS FOR THE GLYCEMIC INDEX DIET

- Cake—cupCake, chocolate, fruit filling or cream filling ☞ 38 (Low)

- Cake—cupCake, chocolate, without icing or filling ☞ 38 (Low)

- Cake—cupCake, not chocolate, icing not specified (average) ☞ 57.5 (Medium)

- Cake—cupCake, not chocolate, with cream and fruit filling ☞ 57.5 (Medium)

- Cake—cupCake, not chocolate, with icing or filling ☞ 57.5 (Medium)

- Cake—cupCake—not chocolate, without icing or filling ☞ 57.5 (Medium)

- Cake—cupCake—NS as to type or icing ☞ 42 (Low)

- Cake—cupCake—NS as to type, with icing ☞ 42 (Low)

- Cake—Dobos Torte (non-chocolate layer cake with chocolate filling and icing) ☞ 38 (Low)

- Cake—frozen yogurt and cake layer, chocolate, with icing ☞ 49.5 (Low)

- Cake—fruit Cake—light or dark, holiday type cake ☞ 57.9 (Medium)

- Cake—German chocolate, with icing and filling ☞ 38 (Low)

- Cake—gingerbread, without icing ☞ 57.9 (Medium)

- Cake—ice cream and cake roll, chocolate ☞ 49.5 (Low)

- Cake—ice cream and cake roll, not chocolate ☞ 51.5 (Low)

- Cake—lemon, low-fat, with icing ☞ 42 (Low)

- Cake—lemon, low-fat, without icing ☞ 42 (Low)

- Cake—lemon, NS as to icing ☞ 42 (Low)

- Cake—lemon, with icing ☞ 42 (Low)

- Cake—lemon, without icing ☞ 42 (Low)
- Cake—marble, with icing ☞ 40 (Low)
- Cake—marble, without icing ☞ 40 (Low)
- Cake—NS as to type, with or without icing ☞ 42 (Low)
- Cake—nut, NS as to icing ☞ 42 (Low)
- Cake—nut, with icing ☞ 42 (Low)
- Cake—nut, without icing ☞ 42 (Low)
- Cake—plum pudding ☞ 57.9 (Medium)
- Cake—poppyseed, without icing ☞ 42 (Low)
- Cake—pound, chocolate ☞ 54 (Low)
- Cake—pound, chocolate, fat free, cholesterol free ☞ 54 (Low)
- Cake—pound, fat free, cholesterol free ☞ 54 (Low)
- Cake—pound, reduced fat, cholesterol free ☞ 54 (Low)
- Cake—pound, with icing ☞ 54 (Low)
- Cake—pound, without icing ☞ 54 (Low)
- Cake—pumpkin, NS as to icing ☞ 62 (Medium)
- Cake—pumpkin, with icing ☞ 62 (Medium)
- Cake—pumpkin, without icing ☞ 62 (Medium)
- Cake—raisin-nut, without icing ☞ 54 (Low)
- Cake—spice, NS as to icing ☞ 42 (Low)
- Cake—spice, with icing ☞ 42 (Low)
- Cake—spice, without icing ☞ 42 (Low)
- Cake—sponge, with icing ☞ 46 (Low)

THE ESSENTIAL FOODS LISTS FOR THE GLYCEMIC INDEX DIET

- Cake—sponge, without icing ► 46 (Low)

- Cake—upside down (all fruits) ► 44 (Low)

- Cake—white, made from home recipe or purchased ready-to-eat, NS as to icing ► 42 (Low)

- Cake—white, pudding-type mix (oil, egg whites, and water added to dry mix), NS as to icing ► 42 (Low)

- Cake—white, pudding-type mix (oil, egg whites, and water added to dry mix), with icing ► 42 (Low)

- Cake—white, pudding-type mix (oil, egg whites, and water added to dry mix), without icing ► 42 (Low)

- Cake—white, standard-type mix (egg whites and water added to mix), with icing ► 42 (Low)

- Cake—white, standard-type mix (egg whites and water added to mix), without icing ► 42 (Low)

- Cake—white, standard-type mix (egg whites and water added), NS as to icing ► 42 (Low)

- Cake—white, with icing, made from home recipe or purchased ready-to-eat ► 42 (Low)

- Cake—white, without icing, made from home recipe or purchased ready-to-eat ► 42 (Low)

- Cake—yellow, made from home recipe or purchased ready-to-eat, NS as to icing ► 42 (Low)

- Cake—yellow, pudding-type mix (oil, eggs, and water added to dry mix), NS as to icing ► 42 (Low)

- Cake—yellow, pudding-type mix (oil, eggs, and water added to dry mix), with icing ► 42 (Low)

- Cake—yellow, pudding-type mix (oil, eggs, and water added to dry mix), without icing ► 42 (Low)

- Cake—yellow, standard-type mix (eggs and water added to dry mix), NS as to icing ☛ 42 (Low)

- Cake—yellow, standard-type mix (eggs and water added to dry mix), with icing ☛ 42 (Low)

- Cake—yellow, standard-type mix (eggs and water added to dry mix), without icing ☛ 42 (Low)

- Cake—yellow, with icing, made from home recipe or purchased ready-to-eat ☛ 42 (Low)

- Cake—yellow, without icing, made from home recipe or purchased ready-to-eat ☛ 42 (Low)

- Cake—zucchini, with icing ☛ 57.9 (Medium)

- Cake—zucchini, without icing ☛ 57.9 (Medium)

- Cheesecake—Common ☛ 50 (Low)

- Cheesecake—with fruit ☛ 50 (Low)

- Cheesecake—chocolate ☛ 50 (Low)

- Cheesecake—chocolate, low fat ☛ 50 (Low)

- Cheesecake—diet ☛ 50 (Low)

- Cheesecake—diet, made with fruit ☛ 50 (Low)

- Cobbler—apple from frozen ☛ 46 (Low)

- Cobbler—apple from fresh ☛ 46 (Low)

- Cobbler—berry ☛ 59 (Medium)

- Cobbler—cherry ☛ 55 (Low)

- Cobbler—peach ☛ 55 (Low)

- Cobbler—pineapple ☛ 59 (Medium)

- Cobbler—Apple Pomegranate ☛ 51 (Low)

THE ESSENTIAL FOODS LISTS FOR THE GLYCEMIC INDEX DIET

- Cobbler—Plum ☛ 58 (Medium)
- Cobbler—Blueberry ☛ 56 (Medium)
- Cobbler—Peach-Lavender ☛ 58 (Medium)
- Cobbler—Strawberry Buttermilk ☛ 57 (Medium)
- Cobbler—Mixed-Fruit ☛ 59 (Medium)
- Cobbler—Peach Apricot ☛ 57 (Medium)
- Coffee cake—crumb ☛ 58 (Medium)
- Coffee cake—crumb cheese-filled ☛ 58 (Medium)
- Coffee cake—quick-bread type or crumb, custard filled ☛ 58 (Medium)
- Coffee cake—crumb, low fat, cholesterol-free ☛ 58 (Medium)
- Coffee cake—crumb, with fruit ☛ 58 (Medium)
- Coffee cake—crumb, with icing ☛ 58 (Medium)
- Coffee cake—Common ☛ 58 (Medium)
- Coffee cake—yeast type ☛ 58 (Medium)
- Coffee cake—yeast type, fat-free, prepared with fruit ☛ 58 (Medium)
- Coffee cake—yeast type, purchased at a bakery ☛ 58 (Medium)
- Coffee cake—yeast type, prepared from home recipe ☛ 58 (Medium)
- Cream puff, eclair, custard or cream filled, iced ☛ 59 (Medium)
- Cream puff, eclair, custard or cream filled, iced, reduced fat ☛ 59 (Medium)
- Cream puff, eclair, custard or cream filled, not iced ☛ 59 (Medium)

- Cream puff, eclair, custard or cream filled, NS as to icing ➤ 59 (Medium)

- Crepe, plain ➤ 67 (Medium)

- Crisp, apple, apple dessert ➤ 48.7 (Low)

- Crisp, cherry ➤ 59 (Medium)

- Crisp, peach ➤ 59 (Medium)

- Crisp, rhubarb ➤ 59 (Medium)

- Crispbread, rye, no added fat ➤ 64 (Medium)

- Crispbread, wheat or rye, extra crispy ➤ 64 (Medium)

- Crispbread, wheat, no added fat ➤ 55 (Medium)

- Croissant ➤ 67 (Medium)

- Croissant, cheese ➤ 67 (Medium)

- Croissant, chocolate ➤ 67 (Medium)

- Croissant, fruit ➤ 67 (Medium)

- Crumpet ➤ 69 (Medium)

- Crumpet, toasted ➤ 69 (Medium)

- Danish pastry, plain or spice ➤ 59 (Medium)

- Danish pastry, with cheese ➤ 59 (Medium)

- Danish pastry, with cheese, fat free, cholesterol free ➤ 59 (Medium)

- Danish pastry, with fruit ➤ 59 (Medium)

- Danish pastry, with nuts ➤ 59 (Medium)

- Empanada—Mexican style, pumpkin ➤ 59 (Medium)

- French toast sticks, plain ➤ 67 (Medium)

THE ESSENTIAL FOODS LISTS FOR THE GLYCEMIC INDEX DIET

- French toast, plain ☞ 67 (Medium)
- Fritter, apple ☞ 59 (Medium)
- Muffin—bran with fruit, low-fat ☞ 60 (Medium)
- Muffin—bran with fruit, no fat, no cholesterol ☞ 60 (Medium)
- Muffin—carrot ☞ 62 (Medium)
- Muffin—chocolate ☞ 53 (Low)
- Muffin—chocolate chip ☞ 53 (Low)
- Muffin—English, multigrain ☞ 43 (Low)
- Muffin—English, multigrain, toasted ☞ 43 (Low)
- Muffin—English, oat bran, toasted ☞ 47 (Low)
- Muffin—fruit and/or nuts ☞ 59 (Medium)
- Muffin—fruit, fat free, cholesterol free ☞ 59 (Medium)
- Muffin—multigrain, with nuts ☞ 64.5 (Medium)
- Muffin—Common ☞ 61.1 (Medium)
- Muffin—oat bran ☞ 60 (Medium)
- Muffin—oat bran with fruit and/or nuts ☞ 60 (Medium)
- Muffin—oatmeal ☞ 69 (Medium)
- Muffin—plain ☞ 44 (Low)
- Muffin—pumpkin ☞ 62 (Medium)
- Muffin—wheat ☞ 60 (Medium)
- Muffin—wheat bran ☞ 60 (Medium)
- Muffin—whole wheat ☞ 60 (Medium)
- Muffin—zucchini ☞ 57.9 (Medium)

- Pancakes—cornmeal ☞ 67 (Medium)

- Pancakes—plain ☞ 67 (Medium)

- Pancakes—reduced calorie, high fiber ☞ 67 (Medium)

- Pancakes—sour dough ☞ 67 (Medium)

- Pancakes—whole-wheat ☞ 67 (Medium)

- Pancakes—with fruit ☞ 67 (Medium)

- Pastry—fruit-filled ☞ 59 (Medium)

- Pastry—Italian, with cheese ☞ 59 (Medium)

- Pastry—mainly flour, almond and water, fried ☞ 59 (Medium)

- Pastry—mainly flour and water, fried ☞ 59 (Medium)

- Pastry—Oriental, prepared with almond paste filling, fried ☞ 59 (Medium)

- Pastry—Oriental, prepared with almond paste filling, baked ☞ 59 (Medium)

- Pastry—Oriental, prepared with bean paste, fried ☞ 59 (Medium)

- Pastry—Oriental, prepared with bean paste, baked ☞ 59 (Medium)

- Pastry—puff ☞ 59 (Medium)

- Pastry—puff, custard or cream filled, icing not specified ☞ 59 (Medium)

- Pie—apple, diet ☞ 59 (Medium)

- Pie—apple, fried ☞ 59 (Medium)

- Pie—apple ☞ 59 (Medium)

- Pie—apple, one crust ☞ 59 (Medium)

- Pie—apple, two crusts ☞ 59 (Medium)

THE ESSENTIAL FOODS LISTS FOR THE GLYCEMIC INDEX DIET

- Pie—apricot, fried ☞ 59 (Medium)
- Pie—apricot, two crusts ☞ 59 (Medium)
- Pie—banana cream ☞ 59 (Medium)
- Pie—berry ☞ 59 (Medium)
- Pie—blackberry, two crusts ☞ 59 (Medium)
- Pie—blueberry ☞ 59 (Medium)
- Pie—blueberry, one crust ☞ 59 (Medium)
- Pie—blueberry, two crusts ☞ 59 (Medium)
- Pie—buttermilk ☞ 59 (Medium)
- Pie—cherry, fried ☞ 59 (Medium)
- Pie—cherry ☞ 59 (Medium)
- Pie—cherry, prepared with sour cream and/or cream cheese ☞ 59 (Medium)
- Pie—cherry, one crust ☞ 59 (Medium)
- Pie—cherry, two crusts ☞ 59 (Medium)
- Pie—chess ☞ 59 (Medium)
- Pie—chocolate cream ☞ 59 (Medium)
- Pie—chocolate cream ☞ 59 (Medium)
- Pie—chocolate marshmallow ☞ 59 (Medium)
- Pie—coconut cream ☞ 59 (Medium)
- Pie—coconut cream ☞ 59 (Medium)
- Pie—custard ☞ 59 (Medium)
- Pie—individual size or tart ☞ 59 (Medium)
- Pie—lemon (not cream) ☞ 59 (Medium)

- Pie—lemon (not merinue) ☞ 59 (Medium)
- Pie—lemon cream ☞ 59 (Medium)
- Pie—lemon meringue ☞ 59 (Medium)
- Pie—mince ☞ 59 (Medium)
- Pie—mince, two crusts ☞ 59 (Medium)
- Pie—Common ☞ 59 (Medium)
- Pie—oatmeal ☞ 59 (Medium)
- Pie—peach, fried ☞ 59 (Medium)
- Pie—peach ☞ 59 (Medium)
- Pie—peach, one crust ☞ 59 (Medium)
- Pie—peach, two crusts ☞ 59 (Medium)
- Pie—peanut butter cream ☞ 59 (Medium)
- Pie—pecan ☞ 59 (Medium)
- Pie—pineapple cream ☞ 59 (Medium)
- Pie—pineapple ☞ 59 (Medium)
- Pie—pineapple, two crusts ☞ 59 (Medium)
- Pie—plum, two crusts ☞ 59 (Medium)
- Pie—praline mousse ☞ 59 (Medium)
- Pie—prune, one crust ☞ 59 (Medium)
- Pie—pudding ☞ 59 (Medium)
- Pie—pudding, with chocolate coating ☞ 59 (Medium)
- Pie—pumpkin ☞ 59 (Medium)
- Pie—raisin ☞ 59 (Medium)

THE ESSENTIAL FOODS LISTS FOR THE GLYCEMIC INDEX DIET

- Pie—raisin, two crusts ☛ 59 (Medium)
- Pie—raspberry, one crust ☛ 59 (Medium)
- Pie—raspberry, two crusts ☛ 59 (Medium)
- Pie—rhubarb, one crust ☛ 59 (Medium)
- Pie—rhubarb, two crusts ☛ 59 (Medium)
- Pie—squash ☛ 59 (Medium)
- Pie—strawberry cream ☛ 59 (Medium)
- Pie—strawberry, one crust ☛ 59 (Medium)
- Pie—strawberry rhubarb, two crusts ☛ 59 (Medium)
- Pie—sweetpotato ☛ 59 (Medium)
- Pie—vanilla cream ☛ 59 (Medium)
- Roll—multigrain ☛ 43 (Low)
- Roll—multigrain, toasted ☛ 43 (Low)
- Roll—pumpernickel ☛ 50 (Low)
- Roll—pumpernickel, toasted ☛ 50 (Low)
- Roll—rye ☛ 58 (Medium)
- Roll—sour dough ☛ 54 (Low)
- Roll—sweet ☛ 57.9 (Medium)
- Roll—sweet, cinnamon bun, frosted ☛ 57.9 (Medium)
- Roll—sweet, cinnamon bun, no frosting ☛ 57.9 (Medium)
- Roll—sweet, crumb topping, Mexican (Pan Dulce) ☛ 59 (Medium)
- Roll—sweet, no topping, Mexican (Pan Dulce) ☛ 59 (Medium)
- Roll—sweet, sugar topping, Mexican (Pan Dulce) ☛ 59 (Medium)

- Roll—sweet, toasted ☛ 57.9 (Medium)
- Roll—sweet, with fruit and nuts, frosted ☛ 57.9 (Medium)
- Roll—sweet, with fruit, frosted ☛ 57.9 (Medium)
- Roll—sweet, with fruit, frosted, diet ☛ 57.9 (Medium)
- Roll—sweet, with fruit, frosted, fat free ☛ 57.9 (Medium)
- Roll—sweet, with fruit, no frosting ☛ 57.9 (Medium)
- Roll—sweet, with nuts, frosted ☛ 57.9 (Medium)
- Roll—sweet, with nuts, no frosting ☛ 57.9 (Medium)
- Roll—white, soft, and/or high fiber ☛ 68 (Medium)
- Roll—white, soft, and/or high fiber, toasted ☛ 68 (Medium)
- Sopaipilla—without syrup or honey ☛ 59 (Medium)
- Strudel—apple ☛ 59 (Medium)
- Strudel—berry ☛ 59 (Medium)
- Strudel—cherry ☛ 59 (Medium)
- Strudel—fruits ☛ 59 (Medium)
- Tamale—sweet, with fruit ☛ 59 (Medium)
- Turnover or dumpling—apple ☛ 59 (Medium)
- Turnover or dumpling—berry ☛ 59 (Medium)
- Turnover or dumpling—cherry ☛ 59 (Medium)
- Turnover or dumpling—lemon ☛ 59 (Medium)
- Turnover or dumpling—peach ☛ 59 (Medium)
- Turnover or dumpling—guava ☛ 59 (Medium)

13

DAIRY AND ALTERNATIVES: LOW AND MEDIUM GLYCEMIC INDEX FOODS

- Butter-margarine blend, salted ☛ 50 (Low)
- Butter-margarine blend, unsalted ☛ 50 (Low)
- Butter-vegetable oil blend ☛ 50 (Low)
- Butter—Light, stick, salted ☛ 0 (Low)
- Butter—Light, stick, unsalted ☛ 0 (Low)
- Butter—Light, whipped, tub, salted ☛ 0 (Low)
- Butter, minimally processed ☛ 50 (Low)
- Butter, stick, salted ☛ 50 (Low)
- Butter, stick, unsalted ☛ 50 (Low)
- Butter, whipped, stick, salted ☛ 50 (Low)
- Butter, whipped, tub, salted ☛ 50 (Low)
- Butter, whipped, tub, unsalted ☛ 50 (Low)
- Buttermilk, fluid, 2% fat ☛ 29.5 (Low)

- Buttermilk, fluid, nonfat ☛ 32 (Low)
- Carry-out milk shake, chocolate ☛ 44 (Low)
- Carry-out milk shake, flavors other than chocolate ☛ 44 (Low)
- Cheese—cottage, minimally processed ☛ 29.5 (Low)
- Cheese—cottage, salted, dry curd ☛ 32 (Low)
- Cheese—cottage, with fruit ☛ 42.5 (Low)
- Cheese—cream ☛ 27 (Low)
- Cheese—cream, low-fat ☛ 27 (Low)
- Cheese—Feta ☛ 27 (Low)
- Cheese—Fontina ☛ 27 (Low)
- Cheese—goat ☛ 27 (Low)
- Cheese—Limburger ☛ 27 (Low)
- Cheese—Monterey ☛ 27 (Low)
- Cheese—Mozzarella, low sodium ☛ 27 (Low)
- Cheese—Mozzarella, average value ☛ 27 (Low)
- Cheese—Mozzarella, nonfat or fat free ☛ 32 (Low)
- Cheese—Mozzarella, part skim ☛ 27 (Low)
- Cheese—Muenster ☛ 27 (Low)
- Cheese—Muenster, low-fat ☛ 27 (Low)
- Cheese—natural, Cheddar or American type ☛ 27 (Low)
- Cheese—natural, minimally processed ☛ 27 (Low)
- Cheese—minimally processed ☛ 27 (Low)
- Cheese—Parmesan, dry grated ☛ 27 (Low)

THE ESSENTIAL FOODS LISTS FOR THE GLYCEMIC INDEX DIET

- Cheese—Parmesan, hard ☛ 27 (Low)
- Cheese—Parmesan, low sodium ☛ 27 (Low)
- Cheese—processed cheese common ☛ 27 (Low)
- Cheese—processed cheese, American type based ☛ 27 (Low)
- Cheese—processed cheese, Cheddar based ☛ 27 (Low)
- Cheese—processed cheese, Swiss based ☛ 27 (Low)
- Cheese—processed cream cheese ☛ 32 (Low)
- Cheese—processed, American and Swiss cheese based ☛ 27 (Low)
- Cheese—processed, American or Cheddar type based low fat ☛ 27 (Low)
- Cheese—processed, American or Cheddar type based, fat free ☛ 32 (Low)
- Cheese—processed, American or Cheddar type based, low sodium ☛ 27 (Low)
- Cheese—processed, American or Cheddar type based, reduced fat ☛ 27 (Low)
- Cheese—processed, made with vegetables ☛ 27 (Low)
- Cheese—processed, Mozzarella based, low sodium ☛ 27 (Low)
- Cheese—processed, Swiss cheese-based ☛ 27 (Low)
- Cheese—processed, Swiss cheese-based, low sodium ☛ 27 (Low)
- Cheese—processed, Swiss cheese-based, low-fat ☛ 27 (Low)
- Cheese—processed, Swiss cheese-based, low-fat, low sodium ☛ 27 (Low)
- Cheese—processed, Colby, based low fat, low sodium ☛ 27 (Low)
- Cheese—Provolone ☛ 27 (Low)

- Cheese—Provolone, reduced fat, and/or reduced-sodium ☞ 27 (Low)
- Cheese—Ricotta ☞ 27 (Low)
- Cheese—Semi-soft, low sodium ☞ 27 (Low)
- Cheese—Swiss ☞ 27 (Low)
- Cheese—Swiss, low sodium ☞ 27 (Low)
- Cheese—Swiss, low-fat ☞ 27 (Low)
- Cheese—yogurt, common ☞ 27 (Low)
- Cream substitute—frozen ☞ 27 (Low)
- Cream substitute—frozen, liquid, and/or powdered ☞ 27 (Low)
- Cream substitute—light, liquid ☞ 27 (Low)
- Cream substitute—light, powdered ☞ 27 (Low)
- Cream substitute—liquid ☞ 27 (Low)
- Cream substitute—powdered ☞ 27 (Low)
- Cream—average value, half and half ☞ 27 (Low)
- Cream—half and half ☞ 27 (Low)
- Cream—heavy, fluid ☞ 27 (Low)
- Cream—heavy, whipped and lightly sweetened ☞ 55.4 (Medium)
- Cream—light, fluid ☞ 27 (Low)
- Cream—light, whipped, and unsweetened ☞ 27 (Low)
- Cream—whipped, purchased as pressurized container ☞ 55.4 (Medium)
- Custard industrially made ☞ 38 (Low)
- Custard—Puerto Rican style ☞ 38 (Low)

THE ESSENTIAL FOODS LISTS FOR THE GLYCEMIC INDEX DIET

- Dip—cream cheese base ☞ 27 (Low)
- Dip—sour cream base ☞ 27 (Low)
- Dip—sour cream base, low-calorie ☞ 27 (Low)
- Dip, cheese—chili con queso ☞ 27 (Low)
- Ice cream—average value ☞ 61 (Medium)
- Ice cream—bar or stick, not covered by chocolate ☞ 61 (Medium)
- Ice cream—regular, chocolate ☞ 61 (Medium)
- Ice cream—regular, flavors other than chocolate ☞ 61 (Medium)
- Ice cream—rich, chocolate ☞ 37 (Low)
- Ice cream—rich, flavors other than chocolate ☞ 38 (Low)
- Ice cream—soda, chocolate ☞ 59.5 (Medium)
- Ice cream—soda, flavors other than chocolate ☞ 64.5 (Medium)
- Ice cream—soft serve, average value ☞ 61 (Medium)
- Ice cream—soft serve, chocolate ☞ 61 (Medium)
- Ice cream—soft serve, flavors other than chocolate ☞ 61 (Medium)
- Ice cream—with sherbet ☞ 51.5 (Low)
- Imitation cheese—American type ☞ 27 (Low)
- Imitation cheese—cheddar ☞ 27 (Low)
- Imitation cheese—Edam ☞ 27 (Low)
- Imitation cheese—Mozzarella ☞ 27 (Low)
- Light ice cream—chocolate ☞ 50 (Low)
- Light ice cream—flavors other than chocolate ☞ 50 (Low)
- Light ice cream—fudgesicle ☞ 50 (Low)

- Light ice cream—(average value) ☛ 50 (Low)
- Light ice cream—premium, chocolate ☛ 50 (Low)
- Light ice cream—premium, flavors other than chocolate ☛ 50 (Low)
- Light ice cream—soft serve, chocolate ☛ 50 (Low)
- Light ice cream—soft serve, flavors other than chocolate ☛ 50 (Low)
- Light ice cream—soft serve, NS as to flavor ☛ 50 (Low)
- Light ice cream—with sherbet ☛ 46 (Low)
- Margarine-based spread—fat free, liquid, salted ☛ 50 (Low)
- Margarine-based spread—fat free, tub, salted ☛ 50 (Low)
- Margarine-based spread—liquid, salted ☛ 0 (Low)
- Margarine-based spread—reduced calorie, about 20% fat, tub, salted ☛ 0 (Low)
- Margarine-based spread—reduced calorie, about 20% fat, tub, unsalted ☛ 0 (Low)
- Margarine-based spread—reduced calorie, about 40% fat, stick, salted ☛ 0 (Low)
- Margarine-based spread—reduced calorie, about 40% fat, tub, salted ☛ 50 (Low)
- Margarine-based spread—stick, salted ☛ 0 (Low)
- Margarine-based spread—stick, unsalted ☛ 0 (Low)
- Margarine-based spread—tub, salted ☛ 0 (Low)
- Margarine-based spread—tub, sweetened ☛ 50 (Low)
- Margarine-based spread—tub, unsalted ☛ 0 (Low)

- Margarine-based spread—whipped, tub, salted ☛ 0 (Low)
- Margarine—common ☛ 0 (Low)
- Margarine—liquid, salted ☛ 0 (Low)
- Margarine—stick, salted ☛ 50 (Low)
- Margarine—stick, unsalted ☛ 50 (Low)
- Margarine—tub, salted ☛ 50 (Low)
- Margarine—tub, unsalted ☛ 50 (Low)
- Margarine—whipped, stick, salted ☛ 50 (Low)
- Margarine—whipped, tub, salted ☛ 50 (Low)
- Margarine—whipped, tub, unsalted ☛ 50 (Low)
- Milk beverage—nonfat dry milk , flavors other than chocolate and low-calorie sweetener ☛ 24 (Low)
- Milk beverage—nonfat dry milk, chocolate and low-calorie sweetener ☛ 24 (Low)
- Milk beverage—whole milk, flavors other than chocolate ☛ 35 (Low)
- Milk dessert—frozen, chocolate (no butterfat) ☛ 61 (Medium)
- Milk dessert—frozen, chocolate ☛ 61 (Medium)
- Milk dessert—frozen, flavors other than chocolate ☛ 61 (Medium)
- Milk dessert—frozen, flavors other than chocolate ☛ 61 (Medium)
- Milk dessert—frozen, flavors other than chocolate, low-calorie sweetener ☛ 50 (Low)
- Milk dessert—frozen, flavors other than chocolate, low-fat ☛ 50 (Low)
- Milk dessert—frozen, low-calorie sweetener ☛ 50 (Low)

- Milk dessert—frozen, low-fat, flavors other than chocolate ☞ 50 (Low)
- Milk gravy ☞ 50 (Low)
- Milk shake—average value ☞ 44 (Low)
- Milk shake—common ☞ 44 (Low)
- Milk shake—homemade, chocolate ☞ 44 (Low)
- Milk shake—homemade, chocolate ☞ 44 (Low)
- Milk shake—homemade, flavors other than chocolate ☞ 44 (Low)
- Milk shake—homemade, flavors other than chocolate ☞ 44 (Low)
- Milk shake—made with skim milk, chocolate ☞ 46.5 (Low)
- Milk shake—made with skim milk, flavors other than chocolate ☞ 46.5 (Low)
- Milk shake—prepared with skim milk, chocolate ☞ 46.5 (Low)
- Milk shake—prepared with skim milk, flavors other than chocolate ☞ 46.5 (Low)
- Milk shake—with malt ☞ 53 (Low)
- Milk shake—with malt ☞ 53 (Low)
- Milk-based fruit drink ☞ 42.5 (Low)
- Milk—chocolate, average value ☞ 37 (Low)
- Milk—chocolate, reduced fat ☞ 37.5 (Low)
- Milk—chocolate, skim ☞ 37.5 (Low)
- Milk—chocolate, whole ☞ 36 (Low)
- Milk—condensed, diluted, sweetened ☞ 61 (Medium)
- Milk—condensed, sweetened, average value ☞ 61 (Medium)

THE ESSENTIAL FOODS LISTS FOR THE GLYCEMIC INDEX DIET

- Milk—condensed, undiluted, sweetened ☛ 61 (Medium)
- Milk—cow's, calcium fortified, fluid, 1% fat ☛ 32 (Low)
- Milk—cow's, calcium fortified, fluid, skim or nonfat ☛ 32 (Low)
- Milk—cow's, fluid, 0% fat, lactose reduced ☛ 32 (Low)
- Milk—cow's, fluid, 0% fat, lactose reduced, enriched with calcium ☛ 32 (Low)
- Milk—cow's, fluid, 1% fat ☛ 32 (Low)
- Milk—cow's, fluid, 1% fat, acidophilus ☛ 32 (Low)
- Milk—cow's, fluid, 1% fat, lactose reduced ☛ 32 (Low)
- Milk—cow's, fluid, 1% fat, lactose reduced, enriched with calcium ☛ 32 (Low)
- Milk—cow's, fluid, 2% fat ☛ 29.5 (Low)
- Milk—cow's, fluid, 2% fat, acidophilus ☛ 29.5 (Low)
- Milk—cow's, fluid, 2% fat, lactose reduced ☛ 29.5 (Low)
- Milk—cow's, fluid, whole ☛ 27 (Low)
- Milk—dry, reconstituted, 0% fat ☛ 32 (Low)
- Milk—dry, reconstituted, average value ☛ 32 (Low)
- Milk—dry, reconstituted, low-fat ☛ 32 (Low)
- Milk—dry, reconstituted, whole ☛ 27 (Low)
- Milk—evaporated, undiluted ☛ 27 (Low)
- Milk—evaporated, 2% fat, dilution not specified ☛ 27 (Low)
- Milk—evaporated, 2% fat, undiluted ☛ 27 (Low)
- Milk—evaporated, average value for fat content and dilution ☛ 27 (Low)

- Milk—evaporated, skim, undiluted ☛ 32 (Low)
- Milk—evaporated, skim, used in coffee or tea ☛ 32 (Low)
- Milk—evaporated, used in coffee or tea ☛ 27 (Low)
- Milk—evaporated, whole, diluted ☛ 27 (Low)
- Milk—evaporated, whole, NS as to dilution ☛ 27 (Low)
- Milk—evaporated, whole, undiluted ☛ 27 (Low)
- Milk—evaporated, whole, used in coffee or tea ☛ 27 (Low)
- Milk—flavors other than chocolate, whole milk-based ☛ 35 (Low)
- Milk—goat's, fluid, whole ☛ 27 (Low)
- Milk—imitation, fluid, soy based ☛ 40 (Low)
- Milk—malted, fortified, chocolate, made with milk ☛ 45 (Low)
- Milk—malted, fortified, natural flavor, made with milk ☛ 45 (Low)
- Milk—malted, fortified, NS as to flavor, made with milk ☛ 45 (Low)
- Milk—malted, unfortified, NS as to flavor, made with milk ☛ 45 (Low)
- Milk—(average value) ☛ 29.5 (Low)
- Milk—soy, dry, reconstituted, not baby's ☛ 40 (Low)
- Milk—soy, ready-to-drink, not baby's ☛ 40 (Low)
- Milk—vinegar, and sugar dressing ☛ 50 (Low)
- Mousse—chocolate ☛ 34 (Low)
- Mousse—not chocolate ☛ 34 (Low)
- Pudding—canned, chocolate ☛ 44 (Low)

- Pudding—canned, chocolate and non-chocolate flavors combined ☛ 44 (Low)

- Pudding—canned, chocolate, fat free ☛ 44 (Low)

- Pudding—canned, chocolate, reduced fat ☛ 44 (Low)

- Pudding—canned, flavors other than chocolate ☛ 44 (Low)

- Pudding—canned, flavors other than chocolate, fat free ☛ 44 (Low)

- Pudding—canned, flavors other than chocolate, reduced fat ☛ 44 (Low)

- Pudding—canned, low-calorie, containing artificial sweetener, chocolate ☛ 44 (Low)

- Pudding—canned, low-calorie, containing artificial sweetener, flavors other than chocolate ☛ 44 (Low)

- Pudding—canned, tapioca ☛ 62.5 (Medium)

- Pudding—canned, tapioca, fat free ☛ 62.5 (Medium)

- Pudding—chocolate, prepared from dry mix, low-calorie, containing artificial sweetener, milk added ☛ 44 (Low)

- Pudding—chocolate, prepared from dry mix, milk added ☛ 44 (Low)

- Pudding—chocolate, ready-to-eat, low-calorie, containing artificial sweetener, NS as to from dry mix or canned ☛ 44 (Low)

- Pudding—chocolate, ready-to-eat, NS as to from dry mix or canned ☛ 44 (Low)

- Pudding—coconut ☛ 44 (Low)

- Pudding—Common ☛ 44 (Low)

- Pudding—flavors other than chocolate, prepared from dry mix, low-calorie, containing artificial sweetener, milk added ☛ 44 (Low)

Pudding—flavors other than chocolate, prepared from dry mix, milk added ☛ 44 (Low)

Pudding—flavors other than chocolate, ready-to-eat, low-calorie, containing artificial sweetener, NS as to from dry mix or canned ☛ 44 (Low)

Pudding—flavors other than chocolate, ready-to-eat, NS as to from dry mix or canned ☛ 44 (Low)

Pudding—Indian (milk, molasses and cornmeal-based pudding) ☛ 44 (Low)

Pudding—pumpkin ☛ 44 (Low)

Pudding—rice ☛ 54 (Low)

Pudding—rice flour, with nuts (Indian dessert) ☛ 54 (Low)

Pudding—tapioca, made from dry mix, made with milk ☛ 62.5 (Medium)

Pudding—tapioca, made from home recipe, made with milk ☛ 62.5 (Medium)

Pudding—with fruit and vanilla wafers ☛ 59.1 (Medium)

Queso—Anejo (aged cheese) ☛ 27 (Low)

Queso—Asadero ☛ 27 (Low)

Queso—Chihuahua ☛ 27 (Low)

Queso—Fresco ☛ 27 (Low)

Yogurt—chocolate, nonfat milk ☛ 32 (Low)

Yogurt—chocolate, NS as to type of milk ☛ 33 (Low)

Yogurt—frozen, chocolate, low-fat milk ☛ 50 (Low)

Yogurt—frozen, chocolate, nonfat milk ☛ 50 (Low)

- Yogurt—frozen, chocolate, nonfat milk, with low-calorie sweetener ☛ 50 (Low)
- Yogurt—frozen, chocolate, NS as to type of milk ☛ 50 (Low)
- Yogurt—frozen, chocolate, whole milk ☛ 50 (Low)
- Yogurt—frozen, flavors other than chocolate, low-fat milk ☛ 50 (Low)
- Yogurt—frozen, flavors other than chocolate, nonfat milk ☛ 50 (Low)
- Yogurt—frozen, flavors other than chocolate, nonfat milk, with low-calorie sweetener ☛ 50 (Low)
- Yogurt—frozen, flavors other than chocolate, NS as to type of milk ☛ 50 (Low)
- Yogurt—frozen, flavors other than chocolate, whole milk ☛ 50 (Low)
- Yogurt—frozen, flavors other than chocolate, with sorbet or sorbet-coated ☛ 50 (Low)
- Yogurt—frozen, NS as to flavor, low-fat milk ☛ 50 (Low)
- Yogurt—frozen, NS as to flavor, nonfat milk ☛ 50 (Low)
- Yogurt—frozen, NS as to flavor, NS as to type of milk ☛ 50 (Low)
- Yogurt—fruit variety, low-fat milk ☛ 31 (Low)
- Yogurt—fruit variety, nonfat milk ☛ 32 (Low)
- Yogurt—fruit variety, nonfat milk, sweetened with low-calorie sweetener ☛ 19 (Low)
- Yogurt—fruit variety, NS as to type of milk ☛ 33 (Low)
- Yogurt—fruit variety, whole milk ☛ 33 (Low)
- Yogurt—NS as to type of milk or flavor ☛ 33 (Low)

🥛 Yogurt—plain, low-fat milk ☛ 36 (Low)

🥛 Yogurt—plain, nonfat milk ☛ 36 (Low)

🥛 Yogurt—plain, NS as to type of milk ☛ 31.5 (Low)

🥛 Yogurt—plain, whole milk ☛ 36 (Low)

🥛 Yogurt—vanilla, lemon, maple, or coffee flavor, low-fat milk ☛ 27 (Low)

🥛 Yogurt—vanilla, lemon, maple, or coffee flavor, nonfat milk ☛ 32 (Low)

🥛 Yogurt—vanilla, lemon, maple, or coffee flavor, nonfat milk, sweetened with low-calorie sweetener ☛ 19 (Low)

🥛 Yogurt—vanilla, lemon, or coffee flavor, NS as to type of milk ☛ 27 (Low)

🥛 Yogurt—vanilla, lemon, or coffee flavor, whole milk ☛ 27 (Low)

14

FISH AND SEAFOOD: LOW AND MEDIUM GLYCEMIC INDEX FOODS

- Anchovy—canned, oil or water → 0 (Low)
- Anchovy—cooked, average value for cooking method → 0 (Low)
- Carp—baked or broiled → 50 (Low)
- Carp—steamed or poached → 0 (Low)
- Catfish—baked or broiled → 50 (Low)
- Catfish—steamed or poached → 0 (Low)
- Clams—baked or broiled → 50 (Low)
- Clams—canned, oil or water → 50 (Low)
- Clams—raw → 50 (Low)
- Clams—steamed or boiled → 50 (Low)
- Cod—baked or broiled → 50 (Low)
- Cod—steamed or poached → 0 (Low)
- Conch—baked or broiled → 50 (Low)

- 🦀 Crab—baked or broiled ☞ 50 (Low)
- 🦀 Crab—cooked, average for the cooking method ☞ 0 (Low)
- 🦀 Crab—hard shell, steamed ☞ 0 (Low)
- 🦀 Croaker—baked or broiled ☞ 50 (Low)
- 🦀 Croaker—steamed or poached ☞ 0 (Low)
- 🦀 Fish, in general—baked or broiled ☞ 50 (Low)
- 🦀 Fish, in general—canned ☞ 0 (Low)
- 🦀 Fish, in general—smoked ☞ 0 (Low)
- 🦀 Fish, in general—steamed ☞ 0 (Low)
- 🦀 Flounder—baked or broiled ☞ 50 (Low)
- 🦀 Flounder—cooked, average value for cooking method ☞ 50 (Low)
- 🦀 Flounder—steamed or poached ☞ 0 (Low)
- 🦀 Haddock—baked or broiled ☞ 50 (Low)
- 🦀 Haddock—steamed or poached ☞ 0 (Low)
- 🦀 Haddock, cooked, average value for cooking method ☞ 50 (Low)
- 🦀 Herring—baked or broiled ☞ 50 (Low)
- 🦀 Herring—pickled ☞ 50 (Low)
- 🦀 Herring—raw ☞ 0 (Low)
- 🦀 Herring—smoked, kippered ☞ 0 (Low)
- 🦀 Lobster—baked or broiled ☞ 50 (Low)
- 🦀 Lobster—cooked, average value for cooking method ☞ 50 (Low)
- 🦀 Lobster—steamed or boiled ☞ 50 (Low)
- 🦀 Lobster—without shell, steamed or boiled ☞ 50 (Low)

- Mackerel—baked or broiled ☞ 50 (Low)
- Mackerel—canned ☞ 0 (Low)
- Mackerel—cooked, average value for cooking method ☞ 50 (Low)
- Mullet—baked or broiled ☞ 50 (Low)
- Mussels—steamed or poached ☞ 50 (Low)
- Ocean perch—baked or broiled ☞ 50 (Low)
- Ocean perch—raw ☞ 0 (Low)
- Octopus—dried, boiled ☞ 50 (Low)
- Oysters—baked or broiled ☞ 50 (Low)
- Oysters—canned ☞ 50 (Low)
- Oysters—raw ☞ 50 (Low)
- Oysters—smoked ☞ 50 (Low)
- Perch—baked or broiled ☞ 50 (Low)
- Perch—steamed or poached ☞ 0 (Low)
- Pike—baked or broiled ☞ 50 (Low)
- Pompano—baked or broiled ☞ 50 (Low)
- Pompano—raw ☞ 0 (Low)
- Porgy—baked or broiled ☞ 50 (Low)
- Porgy—raw ☞ 0 (Low)
- Porgy—steamed or poached ☞ 0 (Low)
- Roe—cooked ☞ 50 (Low)
- Roe—sturgeon ☞ 50 (Low)
- Salmon—baked or broiled ☞ 50 (Low)

- 🦐 Salmon—canned, oil or water ☞ 0 (Low)
- 🦐 Salmon—smoked ☞ 0 (Low)
- 🦐 Salmon—steamed or poached ☞ 0 (Low)
- 🦐 Salmon, cooked, average value for cooking method ☞ 0 (Low)
- 🦐 Sardines—canned in oil ☞ 0 (Low)
- 🦐 Sardines—cooked ☞ 0 (Low)
- 🦐 Sardines—skinless, boneless, canned in water or oil ☞ 0 (Low)
- 🦐 Scallops—baked or broiled ☞ 50 (Low)
- 🦐 Scallops—steamed or boiled ☞ 50 (Low)
- 🦐 Sea bass—baked or broiled ☞ 50 (Low)
- 🦐 Sea bass—steamed or poached ☞ 0 (Low)
- 🦐 Shark—steamed or poached ☞ 0 (Low)
- 🦐 Shrimp—baked or broiled ☞ 50 (Low)
- 🦐 Shrimp—canned, oil or water ☞ 50 (Low)
- 🦐 Shrimp—steamed or boiled ☞ 50 (Low)
- 🦐 Shrimp,—cooked, average value for cooking method ☞ 50 (Low)
- 🦐 Snails—cooked, average value for cooking method ☞ 50 (Low)
- 🦐 Squid—baked, broiled ☞ 50 (Low)
- 🦐 Squid—canned in oil or water ☞ 50 (Low)
- 🦐 Squid—pickled ☞ 50 (Low)
- 🦐 Squid—steamed or boiled ☞ 50 (Low)
- 🦐 Swordfish—baked or broiled ☞ 50 (Low)
- 🦐 Swordfish—steamed or poached ☞ 0 (Low)

- Swordfish, cooked, average value for cooking method → 50 (Low)
- Trout—baked or broiled → 50 (Low)
- Trout—smoked → 0 (Low)
- Trout—steamed or poached → 0 (Low)
- Tuna—canned, in oil or water → 0 (Low)
- Tuna—canned, in oil → 0 (Low)
- Tuna—canned, in water → 0 (Low)
- Tuna—fresh—baked or broiled → 50 (Low)
- Tuna—fresh—steamed or poached → 0 (Low)
- Tuna—fresh, raw → 0 (Low)
- Whiting—baked or broiled → 50 (Low)

15

FRUITS: LOW AND MEDIUM GLYCEMIC INDEX FOODS

- Apple chips ☛ 38 (Low)
- Apple—baked, Average value for added sweetener ☛ 38 (Low)
- Apple—baked, unsweetened ☛ 38 (Low)
- Apple—baked, with sugar ☛ 44 (Low)
- Apple—candied ☛ 44 (Low)
- Apple—chips ☛ 29 (Low)
- Apple—cooked or canned, with light syrup ☛ 44 (Low)
- Apple—dried, cooked, with sugar ☛ 29 (Low)
- Apple—dried, uncooked ☛ 29 (Low)
- Apple—fried ☛ 38 (Low)
- Apple—raw ☛ 38 (Low)
- Applesauce—stewed apples, Average value ☛ 38 (Low)
- Applesauce—stewed apples, sweetened with low-calorie sweetener ☛ 38 (Low)

THE ESSENTIAL FOODS LISTS FOR THE GLYCEMIC INDEX DIET

- Applesauce—stewed apples, unsweetened ☞ 38 (Low)
- Applesauce—stewed apples, with sugar ☞ 38 (Low)
- Apricot, dried, uncooked ☞ 31 (Low)
- Avocado—raw ☞ 50 (Low)
- Banana—raw ☞ 52 (Low)
- Banana—red, ripe ☞ 52 (Low)
- Banana—ripe, boiled ☞ 52 (Low)
- Banana—ripe, fried ☞ 52 (Low)
- Berries—raw, (average value) ☞ 40 (Low)
- Cantaloupe—raw ☞ 65 (Medium)
- Cherries—frozen ☞ 22 (Low)
- Cherries—sour, red, cooked, unsweetened ☞ 22 (Low)
- Cherries—sweet—raw (Queen Anne, Bing) ☞ 22 (Low)
- Cherries—sweet, cooked or canned, Average value ☞ 22 (Low)
- Cherries—sweet, cooked or canned, drained solids ☞ 22 (Low)
- Cherries—sweet, cooked or canned, in heavy syrup ☞ 22 (Low)
- Cherries—sweet, cooked or canned, in light syrup ☞ 22 (Low)
- Cherries—sweet, cooked or canned, juice pack ☞ 22 (Low)
- Currants—dried ☞ 64 (Medium)
- Currants—raw ☞ 64 (Medium)
- Fig—dried, cooked, with sugar ☞ 61 (Medium)
- Fig—dried, uncooked ☞ 61 (Medium)
- Fig—raw ☞ 61 (Medium)

- Figs—cooked or canned, in light syrup ☞ 61 (Medium)
- Fruit cocktail (no citrus fruits)—raw ☞ 55 (Medium)
- Fruit cocktail or mix (with citrus fruits)—raw ☞ 55 (Medium)
- Fruit cocktail—cooked or canned, Average value ☞ 55 (Medium)
- Fruit cocktail—cooked or canned, drained solids ☞ 55 (Medium)
- Fruit cocktail—cooked or canned, in heavy syrup ☞ 55 (Medium)
- Fruit cocktail—cooked or canned, in light syrup ☞ 55 (Medium)
- Fruit cocktail—cooked or canned, juice pack ☞ 55 (Medium)
- Fruit cocktail—cooked or canned, unsweetened, water pack ☞ 55 (Medium)
- Fruit cocktail—frozen ☞ 55 (Medium)
- Fruit juice bar—frozen, flavor other than orange ☞ 59 (Medium)
- Fruit juice bar—frozen, orange flavor ☞ 59 (Medium)
- Fruit juice bar—frozen, sweetened with low-calorie sweetener, flavors other than orange ☞ 59 (Medium)
- Fruit juice bar—with cream, frozen ☞ 42 (Low)
- Fruit mixture—dried ☞ 38 (Low)
- Fruit, dried—average value, excluding high glycemic fruits ☞ 38 (Low)
- Grapefruit—canned or frozen, Average value ☞ 25 (Low)
- Grapefruit—canned or frozen, in light syrup ☞ 25 (Low)
- Grapefruit—canned or frozen, unsweetened, water pack ☞ 25 (Low)
- Grapefruit—raw ☞ 25 (Low)
- Grapes—American type, slip skin—raw ☞ 46 (Low)

THE ESSENTIAL FOODS LISTS FOR THE GLYCEMIC INDEX DIET

- Grapes—European type, adherent skin—raw ☞ 46 (Low)
- Grapes—raw, Average value for type ☞ 46 (Low)
- Green Banana—cooked (in saltwater) ☞ 38 (Low)
- Green Banana—fried ☞ 30 (Low)
- Green plantain—fried ☞ 39 (Low)
- Green plantains—boiled ☞ 39 (Low)
- Guacamole—with tomatoes ☞ 50 (Low)
- Guacamole—with tomatoes and chili peppers ☞ 50 (Low)
- Guacamole, average value ☞ 50 (Low)
- Honeydew melon—raw ☞ 65 (Medium)
- Honeydew—frozen ☞ 65 (Medium)
- Ice fruit ☞ 59 (Medium)
- Kiwi fruit—raw ☞ 53 (Low)
- Nectarine—raw ☞ 42 (Low)
- Orange—raw ☞ 42 (Low)
- Orange, mandarin—canned or frozen, drained ☞ 42 (Low)
- Orange, mandarin—canned or frozen, in light syrup ☞ 42 (Low)
- Papaya—cooked or canned ☞ 59 (Medium)
- Papaya—green, cooked ☞ 59 (Medium)
- Papaya—raw ☞ 59 (Medium)
- Peach—canned or cooked, in heavy syrup ☞ 58 (Medium)
- Peach—canned or cooked, in light or medium syrup ☞ 52 (Low)
- Peach—cooked or canned ☞ 42 (Low)

- Peach—cooked or canned, Average value ☞ 58 (Medium)
- Peach—cooked or canned, juice pack ☞ 38 (Low)
- Peach—frozen, Average value for added sweetener ☞ 58 (Medium)
- Peach—frozen, unsweetened ☞ 42 (Low)
- Peach—raw ☞ 42 (Low)
- Peach, cooked or canned, unsweetened, water pack ☞ 38 (Low)
- Peach, frozen, with sugar ☞ 58 (Medium)
- Peaches ☞ 38 (Low)
- Pear—cooked or canned ☞ 38 (Low)
- Pear—cooked or canned, Average value ☞ 44 (Low)
- Pear—cooked or canned, in heavy syrup ☞ 44 (Low)
- Pear—cooked or canned, in light syrup ☞ 25 (Low)
- Pear—cooked or canned, juice pack ☞ 44 (Low)
- Pear—Japanese—raw ☞ 38 (Low)
- Pear—raw ☞ 38 (Low)
- PineApple—cooked or canned, Average value ☞ 59 (Medium)
- PineApple—cooked or canned, drained solids ☞ 59 (Medium)
- PineApple—cooked or canned, in heavy syrup ☞ 59 (Medium)
- PineApple—cooked or canned, in light syrup ☞ 59 (Medium)
- PineApple—cooked or canned, juice pack ☞ 59 (Medium)
- PineApple—cooked or canned, unsweetened ☞ 59 (Medium)
- Pineapple—raw ☞ 59 (Medium)
- Plantain—boiled, Average value for green or ripe ☞ 39 (Low)

THE ESSENTIAL FOODS LISTS FOR THE GLYCEMIC INDEX DIET

- Plantain—fried, Average value for green or ripe ☞ 39 (Low)
- Plum—cooked or canned, in heavy syrup ☞ 39 (Low)
- Plum—cooked or canned, in light syrup ☞ 39 (Low)
- Plum—raw ☞ 39 (Low)
- Prune—dried, cooked, unsweetened ☞ 29 (Low)
- Prune—dried, cooked, without sugar ☞ 29 (Low)
- Prune—dried, uncooked ☞ 29 (Low)
- Prune, dried, cooked, Average value ☞ 29 (Low)
- Raisins ☞ 64 (Medium)
- Raisins—cooked ☞ 64 (Medium)
- Sorbet fruit—citrus flavor ☞ 59 (Medium)
- Sorbet fruit—noncitrus flavor ☞ 59 (Medium)
- Strawberries—cooked or canned, Average value ☞ 55 (Low)
- Strawberries—cooked or canned, in syrup ☞ 55 (Low)
- Strawberries—frozen, Average value ☞ 55 (Low)
- Strawberries—frozen, unsweetened ☞ 40 (Low)
- Strawberries—frozen, with sugar ☞ 55 (Low)
- Strawberries—raw ☞ 40 (Low)
- Strawberries—raw, with sugar ☞ 55 (Low)
- Tangelo—raw ☞ 42 (Low)
- Tangerine—raw ☞ 42 (Low)

16

GRAINS: LOW AND MEDIUM GLYCEMIC INDEX FOODS

- Barleypearl ➤ 25 (Low)
- 100% Bran ➤ 42 (Low)
- All-Bran ➤ 42 (Low)
- All-Bran with Extra Fiber ➤ 42 (Low)
- Barley—cooked, with fat ➤ 25 (Low)
- Barley—cooked, without fat ➤ 25 (Low)
- Breakfast bar—date, yogurt coating ➤ 53.5 (Low)
- Breakfast bar—diet ➤ 39.3 (Low)
- Buckwheat groats—cooked, with fat ➤ 45 (Low)
- Buckwheat groats—cooked, without fat ➤ 45 (Low)
- Bulgur—canned, average value ➤ 48 (Low)
- Bulgur—canned, with fat ➤ 48 (Low)
- Bulgur—canned, without fat ➤ 48 (Low)

- Bulgur—cooked or canned, average value ☛ 48 (Low)
- Bulgur—cooked or canned, with fat ☛ 48 (Low)
- Bulgur—cooked or canned, without fat ☛ 48 (Low)
- Corn—canned, yellow, low-sodium, with fat ☛ 46 (Low)
- Corn—canned, yellow, low-sodium, without fat ☛ 46 (Low)
- Corn—cooked, average (fresh, frozen, canned) ☛ 53.5 (Low)
- Corn—cooked, average (fresh, frozen, canned), cream style ☛ 53.5 (Low)
- Corn—cooked, average (fresh, frozen, canned), with cream sauce ☛ 46.2 (Low)
- Corn—cooked, average (fresh, frozen, canned), with fat ☛ 53.5 (Low)
- Corn—cooked, average (fresh, frozen, canned), without fat ☛ 53.5 (Low)
- Corn—from canned cooked, not specified if fat is added ☛ 46 (Low)
- Corn—from canned, cooked, white, average ☛ 46 (Low)
- Corn—from canned, cooked, white, with fat ☛ 46 (Low)
- Corn—from canned, cooked, white, without fat ☛ 46 (Low)
- Corn—from canned, cooked, with fat ☛ 46 (Low)
- Corn—from canned, cooked, without fat ☛ 46 (Low)
- Corn—from canned, cooked, yellow ☛ 46 (Low)
- Corn—from canned, cooked, yellow and white, without fat ☛ 46 (Low)
- Corn—from canned, cooked, yellow, with fat ☛ 46 (Low)

- Corn—from canned, cooked, yellow, without fat ☞ 46 (Low)
- Corn—from canned, white, cream-style ☞ 46 (Low)
- Corn—from canned, yellow, cream-style ☞ 46 (Low)
- Corn—from canned, yellow, with fat, cream-style ☞ 46 (Low)
- Corn—from fresh cooked, fat not added in cooking ☞ 53.5 (Low)
- Corn—from fresh cooked, with fat ☞ 53.5 (Low)
- Corn—from fresh, cooked (average) ☞ 53.5 (Low)
- Corn—from fresh, cooked, cream sauce ☞ 46.2 (Low)
- Corn—from fresh, cooked, white, average ☞ 53.5 (Low)
- Corn—from fresh, cooked, white, with fat ☞ 53.5 (Low)
- Corn—from fresh, cooked, white, without fat ☞ 53.5 (Low)
- Corn—from fresh, cooked, yellow ☞ 53.5 (Low)
- Corn—from fresh, cooked, yellow and white ☞ 53.5 (Low)
- Corn—from fresh, cooked, yellow and white, with fat ☞ 53.5 (Low)
- Corn—from fresh, cooked, yellow and white, without fat ☞ 53.5 (Low)
- Corn—from fresh, cooked, yellow, with fat ☞ 53.5 (Low)
- Corn—from fresh, cooked, yellow, without fat ☞ 53.5 (Low)
- Corn—from frozen, cooked (average) ☞ 47 (Low)
- Corn—from frozen, cooked, cream sauce ☞ 46.2 (Low)
- Corn—from frozen, cooked, white, average ☞ 53.5 (Low)
- Corn—from frozen, cooked, white, with fat ☞ 47 (Low)
- Corn—from frozen, cooked, white, without fat ☞ 47 (Low)

THE ESSENTIAL FOODS LISTS FOR THE GLYCEMIC INDEX DIET

- Corn—from frozen, cooked, with fat ☛ 47 (Low)
- Corn—from frozen, cooked, without fat ☛ 47 (Low)
- Corn—from frozen, cooked, yellow ☛ 47 (Low)
- Corn—from frozen, cooked, yellow and white ☛ 47 (Low)
- Corn—from frozen, cooked, yellow and white, without fat ☛ 47 (Low)
- Corn—from frozen, cooked, yellow, with fat ☛ 47 (Low)
- Corn—from frozen, cooked, yellow, without fat ☛ 47 (Low)
- Corn—raw ☛ 53.5 (Low)
- Corn—white, cooked, average (fresh, frozen, canned) ☛ 53.5 (Low)
- Corn—yellow and white, cooked, with fat ☛ 53.5 (Low)
- Corn—yellow and white, cooked, without fat ☛ 53.5 (Low)
- Corn—yellow, cooked, average value ☛ 53.5 (Low)
- Corn—yellow, cooked, average value, with fat ☛ 53.5 (Low)
- Corn—yellow, cooked, average value, without fat ☛ 53.5 (Low)
- Flavored rice—brown and wild ☛ 54 (Low)
- Flavored rice—mixture ☛ 54.7 (Low)
- Flavored rice—white and wild ☛ 54 (Low)
- Kellogg's—Frosted Flakes ☛ 55 (Low)
- Oat bran—cooked, milk, without fat ☛ 44.2 (Low)
- Oat bran—cooked, with fat ☛ 55 (Low)
- Oat bran—cooked, without fat ☛ 55 (Low)
- Rice—brown and wild, cooked, fat added in cooking ☛ 54 (Low)

🌾 Rice—brown and wild, cooked, fat not added in cooking ➤ 54 (Low)

🌾 Rice—brown and wild, cooked, Not Specified as to fat added in cooking ➤ 54 (Low)

🌾 Rice—brown, cooked, instant, Not Specified as to fat added in cooking ➤ 55 (Low)

🌾 Rice—brown, cooked, regular, fat added in cooking ➤ 55 (Low)

🌾 Rice—brown, cooked, regular, fat not added in cooking ➤ 55 (Low)

🌾 Rice—brown, cooked, regular ➤ 55 (Low)

🌾 Rice—white and wild, cooked, fat added in cooking ➤ 54 (Low)

🌾 Rice—white and wild, cooked, fat not added in cooking ➤ 54 (Low)

🌾 Rice—white and wild, cooked ➤ 54 (Low)

🌾 Rice—white, cooked, converted, fat added in cooking ➤ 47 (Low)

🌾 Rice—white, cooked, converted, fat not added in cooking ➤ 47 (Low)

🌾 Rice—white, cooked, converted ➤ 47 (Low)

17

LEGUMES: LOW AND MEDIUM GLYCEMIC INDEX FOODS

- Baked beans—low sodium ☛ 48 (Low)
- Baked beans—(average value) ☛ 48 (Low)
- Baked beans—with pork and sweet sauce ☛ 48 (Low)
- Baked beans—with tomato sauce ☛ 48 (Low)
- Bayo Beans—dry, cooked ☛ 20 (Low)
- Bayo Beans—dry, cooked, with fat ☛ 20 (Low)
- Bayo Beans—dry, cooked, without fat ☛ 20 (Low)
- Beans green string—with onions, cooked, with fat ☛ 32 (Low)
- Beans lima—immature, canned ☛ 32 (Low)
- Beans lima—immature, cooked ☛ 32 (Low)
- Beans lima—immature, cooked, from canned ☛ 32 (Low)
- Beans lima—immature, cooked, from canned, with fat ☛ 32 (Low)
- Beans lima—immature, cooked, from canned, without fat ☛ 32 (Low)

- Beans lima—immature, cooked, from fresh, with fat ☞ 32 (Low)
- Beans lima—immature, cooked, from fresh, without fat ☞ 32 (Low)
- Beans lima—immature, cooked, from frozen ☞ 32 (Low)
- Beans lima—immature, cooked, from frozen, with fat ☞ 32 (Low)
- Beans lima—immature, cooked, from frozen, without fat ☞ 32 (Low)
- Beans lima—immature, cooked, with fat ☞ 32 (Low)
- Beans lima—immature, cooked, without fat ☞ 32 (Low)
- Beans lima—immature, from frozen, creamed or with cheese sauce ☞ 31 (Low)
- Beans string—cooked, from canned, with fat ☞ 32 (Low)
- Beans string—cooked, from fresh, with fat ☞ 32 (Low)
- Beans string—cooked, from frozen, with fat ☞ 32 (Low)
- Beans string—cooked, with fat ☞ 32 (Low)
- Beans string—green, canned, with fat ☞ 32 (Low)
- Beans string—green, cooked, from canned, with fat ☞ 32 (Low)
- Beans string—green, cooked, from fresh, with fat ☞ 32 (Low)
- Beans string—green, cooked, from frozen, with fat ☞ 32 (Low)
- Beans string—green, cooked, with fat ☞ 32 (Low)
- Beans string—green, raw ☞ 32 (Low)
- Beans string—yellow, cooked, from canned, with fat ☞ 32 (Low)
- Beans string—yellow, cooked, from fresh, with fat ☞ 32 (Low)
- Beans string—yellow, cooked, from frozen, with fat ☞ 32 (Low)
- Beans string—yellow, cooked, with fat ☞ 32 (Low)

THE ESSENTIAL FOODS LISTS FOR THE GLYCEMIC INDEX DIET

- Beans—dry, cooked with ground beef ☛ 48 (Low)
- Beans—dry, cooked with pork ☛ 48 (Low)
- Beans—dry, cooked, average value for added fat ☛ 29 (Low)
- Beans—dry, cooked, with fat ☛ 29 (Low)
- Beans—dry, cooked, with fat ☛ 29 (Low)
- Boston baked beans ☛ 48 (Low)
- Chickpeas— dry, cooked ☛ 28 (Low)
- Chickpeas— dry, cooked, with fat ☛ 28 (Low)
- Chickpeas— dry, cooked, without fat ☛ 28 (Low)
- Chickpeas— stewed with pig's feet, Puerto Rican style (Garbanzos guisados con patitos de cerdo) ☛ 28 (Low)
- Chili Beans ☛ 48 (Low)
- Cowpeas— dry, cooked ☛ 42 (Low)
- Cowpeas— dry, cooked with pork ☛ 42 (Low)
- Cowpeas— dry, cooked, with fat ☛ 42 (Low)
- Cowpeas— dry, cooked, without fat ☛ 42 (Low)
- Green or yellow split peas—dry, cooked ☛ 32 (Low)
- Green or yellow split peas—dry, cooked, without fat ☛ 32 (Low)
- Lentils—dry, cooked ☛ 28 (Low)
- Lentils—dry, cooked, with fat ☛ 28 (Low)
- Lentils—dry, cooked, without fat ☛ 28 (Low)
- Lima Beans—dry, cooked ☛ 31 (Low)
- Lima Beans—dry, cooked, with fat ☛ 31 (Low)
- Lima Beans—dry, cooked, without fat ☛ 31 (Low)

- Lima Beans—Stewed, dry ☞ 31 (Low)
- Lima Beans—Stewed, dry -Habichuelas coloradas guisadas ☞ 28 (Low)
- Mung Beans—with fat ☞ 37 (Low)
- Mung Beans—without fat ☞ 37 (Low)
- Peas, Cowpeas—cooked, from fresh ☞ 42 (Low)
- Pinto Beans—dry, cooked ☞ 39 (Low)
- Pinto Beans—dry, cooked, with fat ☞ 39 (Low)
- Pinto Beans—dry, cooked, without fat ☞ 39 (Low)
- Pork and beans ☞ 48 (Low)
- Red kidney Beans—dry, cooked ☞ 28 (Low)
- Red kidney Beans—dry, cooked, with fat ☞ 28 (Low)
- Red kidney Beans—dry, cooked, without fat ☞ 28 (Low)
- Refried beans ☞ 42 (Low)
- Soybean curd ☞ 16 (Low)
- Soybean curd—breaded, fried ☞ 16 (Low)
- Soybean curd—deep fried ☞ 16 (Low)
- Soybean meal ☞ 16 (Low)
- SoyBeans—cooked, with fat ☞ 16 (Low)
- Soyburger—meatless, without bun ☞ 16 (Low)
- White Beans—dry, cooked ☞ 13 (Low)
- White Beans—dry, cooked, with fat ☞ 13 (Low)
- White Beans—dry, cooked, without fat ☞ 13 (Low)

18

MEATS AND POULTRY: LOW AND MEDIUM GLYCEMIC INDEX FOODS

- Beef-Offal—Heart :braised ☛ GI = 50 (Low)
- Beef-Offal—Heart :Broiled and/or baked ☛ GI = 0 (Low)
- Beef-Offal—Heart :Fried ☛ GI = 0 (Low)
- Beef-Offal—Heart :Stewed ☛ GI = 0 (Low)
- Beef-Offal—Heart ☛ GI = 0.0 (Low)
- Beef—Bacon ☛ GI = 0.0 (Low)
- Beef—blood sausage ☛ GI = 28 (Low)
- Beef—Bologna ☛ GI = 0.0 (Low)
- Beef—Bottom Round :braised ☛ GI = 50 (Low)
- Beef—Bottom Round :Broiled and/or baked ☛ GI = 0 (Low)
- Beef—Bottom Round :Fried ☛ GI = 0 (Low)
- Beef—Bottom Round :Roast ☛ GI = 0 (Low)
- Beef—Bottom Round :Stewed ☛ GI = 0 (Low)

- Beef—Bottom Round ☛ GI = 0.0 (Low)
- Beef—Brain :braised ☛ GI = 50 (Low)
- Beef—Brain :Broiled and/or baked ☛ GI = 0 (Low)
- Beef—Brain :Fried ☛ GI = 0 (Low)
- Beef—Brain :Stewed ☛ GI = 0 (Low)
- Beef—Brain ☛ GI = 0.0 (Low)
- Beef—Brisket :braised ☛ GI = 50 (Low)
- Beef—Brisket :Broiled and/or baked ☛ GI = 0 (Low)
- Beef—Brisket :Fried ☛ GI = 0 (Low)
- Beef—Brisket :Roast ☛ GI = 0 (Low)
- Beef—Brisket :Stewed ☛ GI = 0 (Low)
- Beef—Brisket ☛ GI = 0.0 (Low)
- Beef—Canned corned beef ☛ GI = 0.0 (Low)
- Beef—Chorizo ☛ GI = 28 (Low)
- Beef—Chuck Roast :braised ☛ GI = 50 (Low)
- Beef—Chuck Roast :Broiled and/or baked ☛ GI = 0 (Low)
- Beef—Chuck Roast :Fried ☛ GI = 0 (Low)
- Beef—Chuck Roast :Roast ☛ GI = 0 (Low)
- Beef—Chuck Roast :Stewed ☛ GI = 0 (Low)
- Beef—Chuck Roast ☛ GI = 0.0 (Low)
- Beef—Chuck Steak Varieties Chart :braised ☛ GI = 50 (Low)
- Beef—Chuck Steak Varieties Chart :Broiled and/or baked ☛ GI = 0 (Low)
- Beef—Chuck Steak Varieties Chart :Fried ☛ GI = 0 (Low)

THE ESSENTIAL FOODS LISTS FOR THE GLYCEMIC INDEX DIET

- Beef—Chuck Steak Varieties Chart :Roast ☞ GI = 0 (Low)
- Beef—Chuck Steak Varieties Chart :Stewed ☞ GI = 0 (Low)
- Beef—Chuck Steak Varieties Chart ☞ GI = 0.0 (Low)
- Beef—Cured meats ☞ GI = 0.0 (Low)
- Beef—Cuts of Steak :braised ☞ GI = 50 (Low)
- Beef—Cuts of Steak :Broiled and/or baked ☞ GI = 0 (Low)
- Beef—Cuts of Steak :Fried ☞ GI = 0 (Low)
- Beef—Cuts of Steak :Roast ☞ GI = 0 (Low)
- Beef—Cuts of Steak :Stewed ☞ GI = 0 (Low)
- Beef—Cuts of Steak ☞ GI = 0.0 (Low)
- Beef—Delmonico Steak :braised ☞ GI = 50 (Low)
- Beef—Delmonico Steak :Broiled and/or baked ☞ GI = 0 (Low)
- Beef—Delmonico Steak :Fried ☞ GI = 0 (Low)
- Beef—Delmonico Steak :Roast ☞ GI = 0 (Low)
- Beef—Delmonico Steak :Stewed ☞ GI = 0 (Low)
- Beef—Delmonico Steak ☞ GI = 0.0 (Low)
- Beef—Frankfurter ☞ GI = 28 (Low)
- Beef—Ground ☞ GI = 0.0 (Low)
- Beef—Ham ☞ GI = 0.0 (Low)
- Beef—Hamburger patty ☞ GI = 0.0 (Low)
- Beef—Hanger Steak :braised ☞ GI = 50 (Low)
- Beef—Hanger Steak :Broiled and/or baked ☞ GI = 0 (Low)
- Beef—Hanger Steak :Fried ☞ GI = 0 (Low)

- Beef—Hanger Steak :Roast ☛ GI = 0 (Low)
- Beef—Hanger Steak :Stewed ☛ GI = 0 (Low)
- Beef—Hanger Steak ☛ GI = 0.0 (Low)
- Beef—Kidney :braised ☛ GI = 50 (Low)
- Beef—Kidney :Broiled and/or baked ☛ GI = 0 (Low)
- Beef—Kidney :Fried ☛ GI = 0 (Low)
- Beef—Kidney :Stewed ☛ GI = 0 (Low)
- Beef—Kidney ☛ GI = 0.0 (Low)
- Beef—Liver :braised ☛ GI = 50 (Low)
- Beef—Liver :Broiled and/or baked ☛ GI = 0 (Low)
- Beef—Liver :Fried ☛ GI = 0 (Low)
- Beef—Liver :Stewed ☛ GI = 0 (Low)
- Beef—Liver ☛ GI = 0.0 (Low)
- Beef—Liver sausage ☛ GI = 0.0 (Low)
- Beef—Liverwurst ☛ GI = 28 (Low)
- Beef—Loin Steaks and/or Steak Types :braised ☛ GI = 50 (Low)
- Beef—Loin Steaks and/or Steak Types :Broiled and/or baked ☛ GI = 0 (Low)
- Beef—Loin Steaks and/or Steak Types :Fried ☛ GI = 0 (Low)
- Beef—Loin Steaks and/or Steak Types :Roast ☛ GI = 0 (Low)
- Beef—Loin Steaks and/or Steak Types :Stewed ☛ GI = 0 (Low)
- Beef—Loin Steaks and/or Steak Types ☛ GI = 0.0 (Low)
- Beef—luncheon meat ☛ GI = 28 (Low)
- Beef—Meatball ☛ GI = 0.0 (Low)

THE ESSENTIAL FOODS LISTS FOR THE GLYCEMIC INDEX DIET

- Beef—Mettwurst ► GI = 0.0 (Low)
- Beef—Mock Tender Petite Fillet :braised ► GI = 50 (Low)
- Beef—Mock Tender Petite Fillet :Broiled and/or baked ► GI = 0 (Low)
- Beef—Mock Tender Petite Fillet :Fried ► GI = 0 (Low)
- Beef—Mock Tender Petite Fillet :Roast ► GI = 0 (Low)
- Beef—Mock Tender Petite Fillet :Stewed ► GI = 0 (Low)
- Beef—Mock Tender Petite Fillet ► GI = 0.0 (Low)
- Beef—Pepperoni ► GI = 28 (Low)
- Beef—Prime Rib :braised ► GI = 50 (Low)
- Beef—Prime Rib :Broiled and/or baked ► GI = 0 (Low)
- Beef—Prime Rib :Fried ► GI = 0 (Low)
- Beef—Prime Rib :Roast ► GI = 0 (Low)
- Beef—Prime Rib :Stewed ► GI = 0 (Low)
- Beef—Prime Rib ► GI = 0.0 (Low)
- Beef—Rib Steak Cuts :braised ► GI = 50 (Low)
- Beef—Rib Steak Cuts :Broiled and/or baked ► GI = 0 (Low)
- Beef—Rib Steak Cuts :Fried ► GI = 0 (Low)
- Beef—Rib Steak Cuts :Roast ► GI = 0 (Low)
- Beef—Rib Steak Cuts :Stewed ► GI = 0 (Low)
- Beef—Rib Steak Cuts ► GI = 0.0 (Low)
- Beef—Roasted ► GI = 0.0 (Low)
- Beef—Round Steak Varieties :braised ► GI = 50 (Low)
- Beef—Round Steak Varieties :Broiled and/or baked ► GI =

0 (Low)

- Beef—Round Steak Varieties :Fried ☛ GI = 0 (Low)
- Beef—Round Steak Varieties :Roast ☛ GI = 0 (Low)
- Beef—Round Steak Varieties :Stewed ☛ GI = 0 (Low)
- Beef—Round Steak Varieties ☛ GI = 0.0 (Low)
- Beef—Salami ☛ GI = 28 (Low)
- Beef—Sausage ☛ GI = 0.0 (Low)
- Beef—Sausage, Italian ☛ GI = 0.0 (Low)
- Beef—Short Loin :braised ☛ GI = 50 (Low)
- Beef—Short Loin :Broiled and/or baked ☛ GI = 0 (Low)
- Beef—Short Loin :Fried ☛ GI = 0 (Low)
- Beef—Short Loin :Roast ☛ GI = 0 (Low)
- Beef—Short Loin :Stewed ☛ GI = 0 (Low)
- Beef—Short Loin ☛ GI = 0.0 (Low)
- Beef—Short Ribs :braised ☛ GI = 50 (Low)
- Beef—Short Ribs :Broiled and/or baked ☛ GI = 0 (Low)
- Beef—Short Ribs :Fried ☛ GI = 0 (Low)
- Beef—Short Ribs :Roast ☛ GI = 0 (Low)
- Beef—Short Ribs :Stewed ☛ GI = 0 (Low)
- Beef—Short Ribs ☛ GI = 0.0 (Low)
- Beef—T-Bone Steak :braised ☛ GI = 50 (Low)
- Beef—T-Bone Steak :Broiled and/or baked ☛ GI = 0 (Low)
- Beef—T-Bone Steak :Fried ☛ GI = 0 (Low)

- Beef—T-Bone Steak :Roast ☛ GI = 0 (Low)
- Beef—T-Bone Steak :Stewed ☛ GI = 0 (Low)
- Beef—T-Bone Steak ☛ GI = 0.0 (Low)
- Beef—Tenderloin :braised ☛ GI = 50 (Low)
- Beef—Tenderloin :Broiled and/or baked ☛ GI = 0 (Low)
- Beef—Tenderloin :Fried ☛ GI = 0 (Low)
- Beef—Tenderloin :Roast ☛ GI = 0 (Low)
- Beef—Tenderloin :Stewed ☛ GI = 0 (Low)
- Beef—Tenderloin ☛ GI = 0.0 (Low)
- Beef—Tongue :braised ☛ GI = 50 (Low)
- Beef—Tongue :Broiled and/or baked ☛ GI = 0 (Low)
- Beef—Tongue :Fried ☛ GI = 0 (Low)
- Beef—Tongue :Stewed ☛ GI = 0 (Low)
- Beef—Tongue ☛ GI = 0.0 (Low)
- Beef—Top Sirloin :braised ☛ GI = 50 (Low)
- Beef—Top Sirloin :Broiled and/or baked ☛ GI = 0 (Low)
- Beef—Top Sirloin :Fried ☛ GI = 0 (Low)
- Beef—Top Sirloin :Roast ☛ GI = 0 (Low)
- Beef—Top Sirloin :Stewed ☛ GI = 0 (Low)
- Beef—Top Sirloin ☛ GI = 0.0 (Low)
- Beef—Tri-Tip :braised ☛ GI = 50 (Low)
- Beef—Tri-Tip :Broiled and/or baked ☛ GI = 0 (Low)
- Beef—Tri-Tip :Fried ☛ GI = 0 (Low)

- Beef—Tri-Tip :Stewed ☛ GI = 0 (Low)
- Beef—Tri-Tip ☛ GI = 0.0 (Low)
- Beef—Tripe :braised ☛ GI = 50 (Low)
- Beef—Tripe :Broiled and/or baked ☛ GI = 0 (Low)
- Beef—Tripe :Fried ☛ GI = 0 (Low)
- Beef—Tripe :Stewed ☛ GI = 0 (Low)
- Beef—Tripe ☛ GI = 0.0 (Low)
- Chicken—Backs and Necks :braised ☛ GI = 50 (Low)
- Chicken—Backs and Necks :Broiled and/or baked ☛ GI = 0 (Low)
- Chicken—Backs and Necks :Fried ☛ GI = 0 (Low)
- Chicken—Backs and Necks :Roast ☛ GI = 0 (Low)
- Chicken—Backs and Necks :Stewed ☛ GI = 0 (Low)
- Chicken—Backs and Necks ☛ GI = 0.0 (Low)
- Chicken—Breast ☛ GI = 0.0 (Low)
- Chicken—Breast Fillet Tenderloin :braised ☛ GI = 50 (Low)
- Chicken—Breast Fillet Tenderloin :Broiled and/or baked ☛ GI = 0 (Low)
- Chicken—Breast Fillet Tenderloin :Fried ☛ GI = 0 (Low)
- Chicken—Breast Fillet Tenderloin :Roast ☛ GI = 0 (Low)
- Chicken—Breast Fillet Tenderloin :Stewed ☛ GI = 0 (Low)
- Chicken—Breast Fillet Tenderloin ☛ GI = 0.0 (Low)
- Chicken—Chorizo ☛ GI = 28 (Low)
- Chicken—Drumstick :braised ☛ GI = 50 (Low)
- Chicken—Drumstick :Broiled and/or baked ☛ GI = 0 (Low)

THE ESSENTIAL FOODS LISTS FOR THE GLYCEMIC INDEX DIET

- Chicken—Drumstick :Fried ► GI = 0 (Low)
- Chicken—Drumstick :Roast ► GI = 0 (Low)
- Chicken—Drumstick :Stewed ► GI = 0 (Low)
- Chicken—Drumstick ► GI = 0.0 (Low)
- Chicken—Leg :braised ► GI = 50 (Low)
- Chicken—Leg :Broiled and/or baked ► GI = 0 (Low)
- Chicken—Leg :Fried ► GI = 0 (Low)
- Chicken—Leg :Roast ► GI = 0 (Low)
- Chicken—Leg :Stewed ► GI = 0 (Low)
- Chicken—Leg ► GI = 0.0 (Low)
- Chicken—Liverwurst ► GI = 28 (Low)
- Chicken—Luncheon meat ► GI = 0.0 (Low)
- Chicken—Nuggets ► GI = 46 (Low)
- Chicken—Pepperoni ► GI = 28 (Low)
- Chicken—Salami ► GI = 28 (Low)
- Chicken—Sausage ► GI = 28 (Low)
- Chicken—Tender :braised ► GI = 50 (Low)
- Chicken—Tender :Broiled and/or baked ► GI = 0 (Low)
- Chicken—Tender :Fried ► GI = 0 (Low)
- Chicken—Tender :Roast ► GI = 0 (Low)
- Chicken—Tender :Stewed ► GI = 0 (Low)
- Chicken—Tender ► GI = 0.0 (Low)
- Chicken—Thigh :braised ► GI = 50 (Low)

- Chicken—Thigh :Broiled and/or baked ☛ GI = 0 (Low)
- Chicken—Thigh :Fried ☛ GI = 0 (Low)
- Chicken—Thigh :Roast ☛ GI = 0 (Low)
- Chicken—Thigh :Stewed ☛ GI = 0 (Low)
- Chicken—Thigh ☛ GI = 0.0 (Low)
- Chicken—Wing :braised ☛ GI = 50 (Low)
- Chicken—Wing :Broiled and/or baked ☛ GI = 0 (Low)
- Chicken—Wing :Fried ☛ GI = 0 (Low)
- Chicken—Wing :Roast ☛ GI = 0 (Low)
- Chicken—Wing :Stewed ☛ GI = 0 (Low)
- Chicken—Wing ☛ GI = 0.0 (Low)
- Eggs—Free-Range ☛ GI = 0.0 (Low)
- Eggs—Free-Run ☛ GI = 0.0 (Low)
- Eggs—Organic ☛ GI = 0.0 (Low)
- Eggs—Standard Brown ☛ GI = 0.0 (Low)
- Lamb—Breast :braised ☛ GI = 50 (Low)
- Lamb—Breast :Broiled and/or baked ☛ GI = 0 (Low)
- Lamb—Breast :Fried ☛ GI = 0 (Low)
- Lamb—Breast :Roast ☛ GI = 0 (Low)
- Lamb—Breast :Stewed ☛ GI = 0 (Low)
- Lamb—Breast ☛ GI = 0.0 (Low)
- Lamb—Cutlets :braised ☛ GI = 50 (Low)
- Lamb—Cutlets :Broiled and/or baked ☛ GI = 0 (Low)

- Lamb—Cutlets :Fried ☞ GI = 0 (Low)
- Lamb—Cutlets :Roast ☞ GI = 0 (Low)
- Lamb—Cutlets :Stewed ☞ GI = 0 (Low)
- Lamb—Cutlets ☞ GI = 0.0 (Low)
- Lamb—Leg :braised ☞ GI = 50 (Low)
- Lamb—Leg :Broiled and/or baked ☞ GI = 0 (Low)
- Lamb—Leg :Fried ☞ GI = 0 (Low)
- Lamb—Leg :Roast ☞ GI = 0 (Low)
- Lamb—Leg :Stewed ☞ GI = 0 (Low)
- Lamb—Leg ☞ GI = 0.0 (Low)
- Lamb—Loin :braised ☞ GI = 50 (Low)
- Lamb—Loin :Broiled and/or baked ☞ GI = 0 (Low)
- Lamb—Loin :Fried ☞ GI = 0 (Low)
- Lamb—Loin :Roast ☞ GI = 0 (Low)
- Lamb—Loin :Stewed ☞ GI = 0 (Low)
- Lamb—Loin ☞ GI = 0.0 (Low)
- Lamb—Neck :braised ☞ GI = 50 (Low)
- Lamb—Neck :Broiled and/or baked ☞ GI = 0 (Low)
- Lamb—Neck :Fried ☞ GI = 0 (Low)
- Lamb—Neck :Roast ☞ GI = 0 (Low)
- Lamb—Neck :Stewed ☞ GI = 0 (Low)
- Lamb—Neck ☞ GI = 0.0 (Low)
- Lamb—Rack :braised ☞ GI = 50 (Low)

- Lamb—Rack :Broiled and/or baked ☛ GI = 0 (Low)
- Lamb—Rack :Fried ☛ GI = 0 (Low)
- Lamb—Rack :Roast ☛ GI = 0 (Low)
- Lamb—Rack :Stewed ☛ GI = 0 (Low)
- Lamb—Rack ☛ GI = 0.0 (Low)
- Lamb—Rump :braised ☛ GI = 50 (Low)
- Lamb—Rump :Broiled and/or baked ☛ GI = 0 (Low)
- Lamb—Rump :Fried ☛ GI = 0 (Low)
- Lamb—Rump :Roast ☛ GI = 0 (Low)
- Lamb—Rump :Stewed ☛ GI = 0 (Low)
- Lamb—Rump ☛ GI = 0.0 (Low)
- Lamb—Shank :braised ☛ GI = 50 (Low)
- Lamb—Shank :Broiled and/or baked ☛ GI = 0 (Low)
- Lamb—Shank :Fried ☛ GI = 0 (Low)
- Lamb—Shank :Roast ☛ GI = 0 (Low)
- Lamb—Shank :Stewed ☛ GI = 0 (Low)
- Lamb—Shank ☛ GI = 0.0 (Low)
- Lamb—Shoulder :braised ☛ GI = 50 (Low)
- Lamb—Shoulder :Broiled and/or baked ☛ GI = 0 (Low)
- Lamb—Shoulder :Fried ☛ GI = 0 (Low)
- Lamb—Shoulder :Roast ☛ GI = 0 (Low)
- Lamb—Shoulder :Stewed ☛ GI = 0 (Low)
- Lamb—Shoulder ☛ GI = 0.0 (Low)

THE ESSENTIAL FOODS LISTS FOR THE GLYCEMIC INDEX DIET

- Pork—back ribs :braised ☛ GI = 50 (Low)
- Pork—back ribs :Broiled and/or baked ☛ GI = 0 (Low)
- Pork—back ribs :Fried ☛ GI = 0 (Low)
- Pork—back ribs :Roast ☛ GI = 0 (Low)
- Pork—back ribs :Stewed ☛ GI = 0 (Low)
- Pork—back ribs ☛ GI = 0.0 (Low)
- Pork—Belly :braised ☛ GI = 50 (Low)
- Pork—Belly :Broiled and/or baked ☛ GI = 0 (Low)
- Pork—Belly :Fried ☛ GI = 0 (Low)
- Pork—Belly :Roast ☛ GI = 0 (Low)
- Pork—Belly :Stewed ☛ GI = 0 (Low)
- Pork—Belly ☛ GI = 0.0 (Low)
- Pork—Cutlets :braised ☛ GI = 50 (Low)
- Pork—Cutlets :Broiled and/or baked ☛ GI = 0 (Low)
- Pork—Cutlets :Fried ☛ GI = 0 (Low)
- Pork—Cutlets :Roast ☛ GI = 0 (Low)
- Pork—Cutlets :Stewed ☛ GI = 0 (Low)
- Pork—Cutlets ☛ GI = 0.0 (Low)
- Pork—Garlic Sausages :braised ☛ GI = 50 (Low)
- Pork—Garlic Sausages :Broiled and/or baked ☛ GI = 0 (Low)
- Pork—Garlic Sausages :Fried ☛ GI = 0 (Low)
- Pork—Garlic Sausages :Roast ☛ GI = 0 (Low)
- Pork—Garlic Sausages :Stewed ☛ GI = 0 (Low)

- Pork—Garlic Sausages ▶ GI = 0.0 (Low)
- Pork—Ham :braised ▶ GI = 50 (Low)
- Pork—Ham :Broiled and/or baked ▶ GI = 0 (Low)
- Pork—Ham :Fried ▶ GI = 0 (Low)
- Pork—Ham :Roast ▶ GI = 0 (Low)
- Pork—Ham :Stewed ▶ GI = 0 (Low)
- Pork—Ham ▶ GI = 0.0 (Low)
- Pork—Loin :braised ▶ GI = 50 (Low)
- Pork—Loin :Broiled and/or baked ▶ GI = 0 (Low)
- Pork—Loin :Fried ▶ GI = 0 (Low)
- Pork—Loin :Roast ▶ GI = 0 (Low)
- Pork—Loin :Stewed ▶ GI = 0 (Low)
- Pork—Loin ▶ GI = 0.0 (Low)
- Pork—Rib chops :braised ▶ GI = 50 (Low)
- Pork—Rib chops :Broiled and/or baked ▶ GI = 0 (Low)
- Pork—Rib chops :Fried ▶ GI = 0 (Low)
- Pork—Rib chops :Roast ▶ GI = 0 (Low)
- Pork—Rib chops :Stewed ▶ GI = 0 (Low)
- Pork—Rib chops ▶ GI = 0.0 (Low)
- Pork—Roasts :braised ▶ GI = 50 (Low)
- Pork—Roasts :Broiled and/or baked ▶ GI = 0 (Low)
- Pork—Roasts :Fried ▶ GI = 0 (Low)
- Pork—Roasts :Roast ▶ GI = 0 (Low)

- Pork—Roasts :Stewed ▶ GI = 0 (Low)
- Pork—Roasts ▶ GI = 0.0 (Low)
- Pork—Sausages :braised ▶ GI = 50 (Low)
- Pork—Sausages :Broiled and/or baked ▶ GI = 0 (Low)
- Pork—Sausages :Fried ▶ GI = 0 (Low)
- Pork—Sausages :Roast ▶ GI = 0 (Low)
- Pork—Sausages :Stewed ▶ GI = 0 (Low)
- Pork—Sausages ▶ GI = 0.0 (Low)
- Pork—Shoulder chops :braised ▶ GI = 50 (Low)
- Pork—Shoulder chops :Broiled and/or baked ▶ GI = 0 (Low)
- Pork—Shoulder chops :Fried ▶ GI = 0 (Low)
- Pork—Shoulder chops :Roast ▶ GI = 0 (Low)
- Pork—Shoulder chops :Stewed ▶ GI = 0 (Low)
- Pork—Shoulder chops ▶ GI = 0.0 (Low)
- Pork—Sirloin chops :braised ▶ GI = 50 (Low)
- Pork—Sirloin chops :Broiled and/or baked ▶ GI = 0 (Low)
- Pork—Sirloin chops :Fried ▶ GI = 0 (Low)
- Pork—Sirloin chops :Roast ▶ GI = 0 (Low)
- Pork—Sirloin chops :Stewed ▶ GI = 0 (Low)
- Pork—Sirloin chops ▶ GI = 0.0 (Low)
- Pork—spare ribs :braised ▶ GI = 50 (Low)
- Pork—spare ribs :Broiled and/or baked ▶ GI = 0 (Low)
- Pork—spare ribs :Fried ▶ GI = 0 (Low)

- Pork—spare ribs :Roast ☞ GI = 0 (Low)
- Pork—spare ribs :Stewed ☞ GI = 0 (Low)
- Pork—spare ribs ☞ GI = 0.0 (Low)
- Turkey—Backs and Necks :braised ☞ GI = 50 (Low)
- Turkey—Backs and Necks :Broiled and/or baked ☞ GI = 0 (Low)
- Turkey—Backs and Necks :Fried ☞ GI = 0 (Low)
- Turkey—Backs and Necks :Roast ☞ GI = 0 (Low)
- Turkey—Backs and Necks :Stewed ☞ GI = 0 (Low)
- Turkey—Backs and Necks ☞ GI = 0.0 (Low)
- Turkey—Breast :braised ☞ GI = 50 (Low)
- Turkey—Breast :Broiled and/or baked ☞ GI = 0 (Low)
- Turkey—Breast :Fried ☞ GI = 0 (Low)
- Turkey—Breast :Roast ☞ GI = 0 (Low)
- Turkey—Breast :Stewed ☞ GI = 0 (Low)
- Turkey—Breast ☞ GI = 0.0 (Low)
- Turkey—Breast Fillet Tenderloin :braised ☞ GI = 50 (Low)
- Turkey—Breast Fillet Tenderloin :Broiled and/or baked ☞ GI = 0 (Low)
- Turkey—Breast Fillet Tenderloin :Fried ☞ GI = 0 (Low)
- Turkey—Breast Fillet Tenderloin :Roast ☞ GI = 0 (Low)
- Turkey—Breast Fillet Tenderloin :Stewed ☞ GI = 0 (Low)
- Turkey—Breast Fillet Tenderloin ☞ GI = 0.0 (Low)
- Turkey—Chorizo ☞ GI = 28 (Low)
- Turkey—Drumstick :braised ☞ GI = 50 (Low)

THE ESSENTIAL FOODS LISTS FOR THE GLYCEMIC INDEX DIET

- Turkey—Drumstick :Broiled and/or baked ☛ GI = 0 (Low)
- Turkey—Drumstick :Fried ☛ GI = 0 (Low)
- Turkey—Drumstick :Roast ☛ GI = 0 (Low)
- Turkey—Drumstick :Stewed ☛ GI = 0 (Low)
- Turkey—Drumstick ☛ GI = 0.0 (Low)
- Turkey—Leg :braised ☛ GI = 50 (Low)
- Turkey—Leg :Broiled and/or baked ☛ GI = 0 (Low)
- Turkey—Leg :Fried ☛ GI = 0 (Low)
- Turkey—Leg :Roast ☛ GI = 0 (Low)
- Turkey—Leg :Stewed ☛ GI = 0 (Low)
- Turkey—Leg ☛ GI = 0.0 (Low)
- Turkey—Liverwurst ☛ GI = 28 (Low)
- Turkey—Pepperoni ☛ GI = 28 (Low)
- Turkey—Salami ☛ GI = 28 (Low)
- Turkey—Sausage ☛ GI = 28 (Low)
- Turkey—Tender :braised ☛ GI = 50 (Low)
- Turkey—Tender :Broiled and/or baked ☛ GI = 0 (Low)
- Turkey—Tender :Fried ☛ GI = 0 (Low)
- Turkey—Tender :Roast ☛ GI = 0 (Low)
- Turkey—Tender :Stewed ☛ GI = 0 (Low)
- Turkey—Tender ☛ GI = 0.0 (Low)
- Turkey—Thigh :braised ☛ GI = 50 (Low)
- Turkey—Thigh :Broiled and/or baked ☛ GI = 0 (Low)

- Turkey—Thigh :Fried ☞ GI = 0 (Low)
- Turkey—Thigh :Roast ☞ GI = 0 (Low)
- Turkey—Thigh :Stewed ☞ GI = 0 (Low)
- Turkey—Thigh ☞ GI = 0.0 (Low)
- Turkey—Wing :braised ☞ GI = 50 (Low)
- Turkey—Wing :Broiled and/or baked ☞ GI = 0 (Low)
- Turkey—Wing :Fried ☞ GI = 0 (Low)
- Turkey—Wing :Roast ☞ GI = 0 (Low)
- Turkey—Wing :Stewed ☞ GI = 0 (Low)
- Turkey—Wing ☞ GI = 0.0 (Low)
- Veal-Offal—Heart :braised ☞ GI = 50 (Low)
- Veal-Offal—Heart :Broiled and/or baked ☞ GI = 0 (Low)
- Veal-Offal—Heart :Fried ☞ GI = 0 (Low)
- Veal-Offal—Heart ☞ GI = 0.0 (Low)
- Veal—Bottom Round :braised ☞ GI = 50 (Low)
- Veal—Bottom Round :Broiled and/or baked ☞ GI = 0 (Low)
- Veal—Bottom Round :Fried ☞ GI = 0 (Low)
- Veal—Bottom Round :Roast ☞ GI = 0 (Low)
- Veal—Bottom Round :Stewed ☞ GI = 0 (Low)
- Veal—Bottom Round ☞ GI = 0.0 (Low)
- Veal—Brain :braised ☞ GI = 50 (Low)
- Veal—Brain :Broiled and/or baked ☞ GI = 0 (Low)
- Veal—Brain :Fried ☞ GI = 0 (Low)

THE ESSENTIAL FOODS LISTS FOR THE GLYCEMIC INDEX DIET

- Veal—Brain ☞ GI = 0.0 (Low)
- Veal—Brisket :braised ☞ GI = 50 (Low)
- Veal—Brisket :Broiled and/or baked ☞ GI = 0 (Low)
- Veal—Brisket :Fried ☞ GI = 0 (Low)
- Veal—Brisket :Roast ☞ GI = 0 (Low)
- Veal—Brisket :Stewed ☞ GI = 0 (Low)
- Veal—Brisket ☞ GI = 0.0 (Low)
- Veal—Chuck Roast :braised ☞ GI = 50 (Low)
- Veal—Chuck Roast :Broiled and/or baked ☞ GI = 0 (Low)
- Veal—Chuck Roast :Fried ☞ GI = 0 (Low)
- Veal—Chuck Roast :Roast ☞ GI = 0 (Low)
- Veal—Chuck Roast :Stewed ☞ GI = 0 (Low)
- Veal—Chuck Roast ☞ GI = 0.0 (Low)
- Veal—Chuck Steak Varieties Chart :braised ☞ GI = 50 (Low)
- Veal—Chuck Steak Varieties Chart :Broiled and/or baked ☞ GI = 0 (Low)
- Veal—Chuck Steak Varieties Chart :Fried ☞ GI = 0 (Low)
- Veal—Chuck Steak Varieties Chart :Roast ☞ GI = 0 (Low)
- Veal—Chuck Steak Varieties Chart :Stewed ☞ GI = 0 (Low)
- Veal—Chuck Steak Varieties Chart ☞ GI = 0.0 (Low)
- Veal—Cuts of Steak :braised ☞ GI = 50 (Low)
- Veal—Cuts of Steak :Broiled and/or baked ☞ GI = 0 (Low)
- Veal—Cuts of Steak :Fried ☞ GI = 0 (Low)
- Veal—Cuts of Steak :Roast ☞ GI = 0 (Low)

- Veal—Cuts of Steak :Stewed ☛ GI = 0 (Low)
- Veal—Cuts of Steak ☛ GI = 0.0 (Low)
- Veal—Delmonico Steak :braised ☛ GI = 50 (Low)
- Veal—Delmonico Steak :Broiled and/or baked ☛ GI = 0 (Low)
- Veal—Delmonico Steak :Fried ☛ GI = 0 (Low)
- Veal—Delmonico Steak :Roast ☛ GI = 0 (Low)
- Veal—Delmonico Steak :Stewed ☛ GI = 0 (Low)
- Veal—Delmonico Steak ☛ GI = 0.0 (Low)
- Veal—Hanger Steak :braised ☛ GI = 50 (Low)
- Veal—Hanger Steak :Broiled and/or baked ☛ GI = 0 (Low)
- Veal—Hanger Steak :Fried ☛ GI = 0 (Low)
- Veal—Hanger Steak :Roast ☛ GI = 0 (Low)
- Veal—Hanger Steak :Stewed ☛ GI = 0 (Low)
- Veal—Hanger Steak ☛ GI = 0.0 (Low)
- Veal—Kidney :braised ☛ GI = 50 (Low)
- Veal—Kidney :Broiled and/or baked ☛ GI = 0 (Low)
- Veal—Kidney :Fried ☛ GI = 0 (Low)
- Veal—Kidney ☛ GI = 0.0 (Low)
- Veal—Liver :braised ☛ GI = 50 (Low)
- Veal—Liver :Broiled and/or baked ☛ GI = 0 (Low)
- Veal—Liver :Fried ☛ GI = 0 (Low)
- Veal—Liver ☛ GI = 0.0 (Low)
- Veal—Loin Steaks and/or Steak Types :braised ☛ GI = 50 (Low)

THE ESSENTIAL FOODS LISTS FOR THE GLYCEMIC INDEX DIET

- Veal—Loin Steaks and/or Steak Types :Broiled and/or baked ► GI = 0 (Low)
- Veal—Loin Steaks and/or Steak Types :Fried ► GI = 0 (Low)
- Veal—Loin Steaks and/or Steak Types :Roast ► GI = 0 (Low)
- Veal—Loin Steaks and/or Steak Types :Stewed ► GI = 0 (Low)
- Veal—Loin Steaks and/or Steak Types ► GI = 0.0 (Low)
- Veal—Mock Tender Petite Fillet :braised ► GI = 50 (Low)
- Veal—Mock Tender Petite Fillet :Broiled and/or baked ► GI = 0 (Low)
- Veal—Mock Tender Petite Fillet :Fried ► GI = 0 (Low)
- Veal—Mock Tender Petite Fillet :Roast ► GI = 0 (Low)
- Veal—Mock Tender Petite Fillet :Stewed ► GI = 0 (Low)
- Veal—Mock Tender Petite Fillet ► GI = 0.0 (Low)
- Veal—Prime Rib :braised ► GI = 50 (Low)
- Veal—Prime Rib :Broiled and/or baked ► GI = 0 (Low)
- Veal—Prime Rib :Fried ► GI = 0 (Low)
- Veal—Prime Rib :Roast ► GI = 0 (Low)
- Veal—Prime Rib :Stewed ► GI = 0 (Low)
- Veal—Prime Rib ► GI = 0.0 (Low)
- Veal—Rib Steak Cuts :braised ► GI = 50 (Low)
- Veal—Rib Steak Cuts :Broiled and/or baked ► GI = 0 (Low)
- Veal—Rib Steak Cuts :Fried ► GI = 0 (Low)
- Veal—Rib Steak Cuts :Roast ► GI = 0 (Low)
- Veal—Rib Steak Cuts :Stewed ► GI = 0 (Low)

- Veal—Rib Steak Cuts ☞ GI = 0.0 (Low)
- Veal—Round Steak Varieties :braised ☞ GI = 50 (Low)
- Veal—Round Steak Varieties :Broiled and/or baked ☞ GI = 0 (Low)
- Veal—Round Steak Varieties :Fried ☞ GI = 0 (Low)
- Veal—Round Steak Varieties :Roast ☞ GI = 0 (Low)
- Veal—Round Steak Varieties :Stewed ☞ GI = 0 (Low)
- Veal—Round Steak Varieties ☞ GI = 0.0 (Low)
- Veal—Short Loin :braised ☞ GI = 50 (Low)
- Veal—Short Loin :Broiled and/or baked ☞ GI = 0 (Low)
- Veal—Short Loin :Fried ☞ GI = 0 (Low)
- Veal—Short Loin :Roast ☞ GI = 0 (Low)
- Veal—Short Loin :Stewed ☞ GI = 0 (Low)
- Veal—Short Loin ☞ GI = 0.0 (Low)
- Veal—Short Ribs :braised ☞ GI = 50 (Low)
- Veal—Short Ribs :Broiled and/or baked ☞ GI = 0 (Low)
- Veal—Short Ribs :Fried ☞ GI = 0 (Low)
- Veal—Short Ribs :Roast ☞ GI = 0 (Low)
- Veal—Short Ribs :Stewed ☞ GI = 0 (Low)
- Veal—Short Ribs ☞ GI = 0.0 (Low)
- Veal—T-Bone Steak :braised ☞ GI = 50 (Low)
- Veal—T-Bone Steak :Broiled and/or baked ☞ GI = 0 (Low)
- Veal—T-Bone Steak :Fried ☞ GI = 0 (Low)
- Veal—T-Bone Steak :Roast ☞ GI = 0 (Low)

THE ESSENTIAL FOODS LISTS FOR THE GLYCEMIC INDEX DIET

- Veal—T-Bone Steak :Stewed ► GI = 0 (Low)
- Veal—T-Bone Steak ► GI = 0.0 (Low)
- Veal—Tenderloin :braised ► GI = 50 (Low)
- Veal—Tenderloin :Broiled and/or baked ► GI = 0 (Low)
- Veal—Tenderloin :Fried ► GI = 0 (Low)
- Veal—Tenderloin :Roast ► GI = 0 (Low)
- Veal—Tenderloin :Stewed ► GI = 0 (Low)
- Veal—Tenderloin ► GI = 0.0 (Low)
- Veal—Tongue :braised ► GI = 50 (Low)
- Veal—Tongue :Broiled and/or baked ► GI = 0 (Low)
- Veal—Tongue :Fried ► GI = 0 (Low)
- Veal—Tongue ► GI = 0.0 (Low)
- Veal—Top Sirloin :braised ► GI = 50 (Low)
- Veal—Top Sirloin :Broiled and/or baked ► GI = 0 (Low)
- Veal—Top Sirloin :Fried ► GI = 0 (Low)
- Veal—Top Sirloin :Roast ► GI = 0 (Low)
- Veal—Top Sirloin :Stewed ► GI = 0 (Low)
- Veal—Top Sirloin ► GI = 0.0 (Low)
- Veal—Tri-Tip :braised ► GI = 50 (Low)
- Veal—Tri-Tip :Broiled and/or baked ► GI = 0 (Low)
- Veal—Tri-Tip :Fried ► GI = 0 (Low)
- Veal—Tri-Tip :Roast ► GI = 0 (Low)
- Veal—Tri-Tip :Stewed ► GI = 0 (Low)

- Veal—Tri-Tip ☛ GI = 0.0 (Low)
- Veal—Tripe :braised ☛ GI = 50 (Low)
- Veal—Tripe :Broiled and/or baked ☛ GI = 0 (Low)
- Veal—Tripe :Fried ☛ GI = 0 (Low)
- Veal—Tripe ☛ GI = 0.0 (Low)

19

MIXED MEALS AND CONVENIENCE FOODS

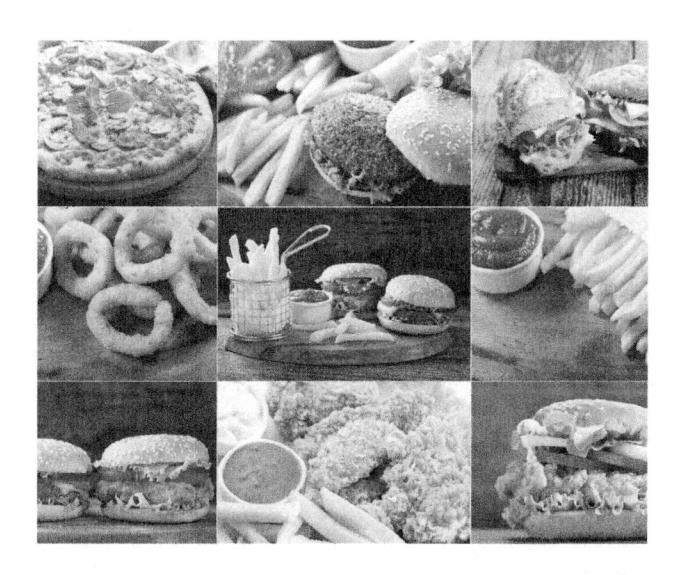

Featuring 250+ more new listings in the category "mixed meals and convenience foods", this essential 2021 reference table provides the GI counts you need to know for generic and brand-name foods. Data were compiled from the most authoritative sources, and some GI values were calculated as the mean of up to five studies.

📖 Bacon—average value concerning meat, cooked ☞ 50 (Low)

📖 Bacon—or side pork, fresh, cooked ☞ 50 (Low)

📖 Bacon—Pork formed, lean meat added, cooked ☞ 50 (Low)

📖 Bacon—Pork NS as to fresh, smoked or cured, cooked ☞ 50 (Low)

📖 Bacon—Pork smoked or cured, cooked ☞ 50 (Low)

📖 Bacon—Pork smoked or cured, cooked, lean only eaten ☞ 50 (Low)

📖 Bacon—Pork smoked or cured, lower sodium ☞ 50 (Low)

📖 Bean soup—home recipe ☞ 64 (Medium)

📖 Bean soup—mixed beans ☞ 64 (Medium)

📖 Bean soup—with bacon or pork ☞ 64 (Medium)

📖 Bean soup—with macaroni ☞ 37.8 (Low)

📖 Bean soup—with macaroni and meat ☞ 38.3 (Low)

📖 Bean soup—with vegetables and rice ☞ 55.3 (Medium)

📖 Beef and noodles—with tomato sauce ☞ 40 (Low)

📖 Beef and rice noodle soup ☞ 53 (Low)

📖 Beef and vegetables—carrots, broccoli, dark-green leafy, soy-based sauce ☞ 49 (Low)

📖 Beef noodle soup ☞ 42 (Low)

📖 Beef noodle soup ☞ 42 (Low)

📖 Beef noodle soup—home recipe ☞ 42 (Low)

📖 Beef noodle soup—home recipe ☞ 42 (Low)

📖 Beef noodle soup—Sopa de carne y fideos ☞ 42 (Low)

- Beef noodle soup—Sopa de carne y fideos ☛ 42 (Low)
- Beef pot pie ☛ 45 (Low)
- Beef pot pie ☛ 45 (Low)
- Beef pot pie ☛ 45 (Low)
- Beef rice soup ☛ 64 (Low)
- Beef rice soup ☛ 64 (Medium)
- Beef sausage— Average Value ☛ 28 (Low)
- Beef sausage— brown and serve, links, cooked ☛ 28 (Low)
- Beef sausage— fresh, bulk, patty or link, cooked ☛ 28 (Low)
- Beef sausage— smoked ☛ 28 (Low)
- Beef sausage— smoked, stick ☛ 28 (Low)
- Beef stew—with potatoes, tomato sauce ☛ 70 (Medium)
- Beef stroganoff soup—chunky style ☛ 42 (Low)
- Beef stroganoff soup—chunky style ☛ 42 (Low)
- Beef stroganoff—with noodles ☛ 46 (Low)
- Beef stroganoff—with noodles ☛ 46 (Low)
- Beef stroganoff—with noodles ☛ 46 (Low)
- Beef vegetable soup—Sopa caldo de Res ☛ 38 (Low)
- Beef vegetable soup—Sopa caldo de Res ☛ 38 (Low)
- Beef vegetable soup—with noodles, stew type, chunky style ☛ 40 (Low)
- Beef vegetable soup—with noodles, stew type, chunky style ☛ 40 (Low)
- Beef vegetable soup—with potato, stew type ☛ 44 (Low)

- Beef vegetable soup—with potato, stew type ☛ 44 (Low)
- Beef vegetable soup—with rice, stew type, chunky style ☛ 51 (Low)
- Beef vegetable soup—with rice, stew type, chunky style ☛ 51 (Low)
- Beef vegetables stew—potatoes, carrots, broccoli, dark-green leafy ☛ 64 (Medium)
- Beef vegetables stew—potatoes, carrots, broccoli, dark-green leafy, tomato sauce ☛ 63 (Medium)
- Beef—sloppy joe without bun ☛ 42 (Low)
- Beef—with barbecue sauce ☛ 38 (Low)
- Beef—with tomato sauce ☛ 37 (Low)
- Beef, bacon— cooked ☛ 50 (Low)
- Beef, bacon— formed, lean meat added, cooked ☛ 50 (Low)
- Beef, rice, and vegetables soup —not carrots, not broccoli ☛ 49 (Low)
- Beef, rice, and vegetables soup —not carrots, not broccoli ☛ 49.1 (Low)
- Beef, rice, and vegetables soup—with carrots, broccoli ☛ 47 (Low)
- Beef, rice, and vegetables soup—with carrots, broccoli ☛ 47.4 (Low)
- Black bean soup ☛ 64 (Medium)
- Black bean soup ☛ 64 (Medium)
- Blood sausage ☛ 28 (Low)
- Bologna ring—smoked ☛ 28 (Low)
- Bologna— Average Value ☛ 28 (Low)

THE ESSENTIAL FOODS LISTS FOR THE GLYCEMIC INDEX DIET

📘 Bologna— beef ☞ 28 (Low)

📘 Bologna— beef and pork, low-fat ☞ 28 (Low)

📘 Bologna— beef, lower sodium ☞ 28 (Low)

📘 Bologna— beef, low-fat ☞ 28 (Low)

📘 Bologna— chicken, beef, and pork ☞ 28 (Low)

📘 Bologna— Lebanon ☞ 28 (Low)

📘 Bologna— pork ☞ 28 (Low)

📘 Bologna— pork and beef ☞ 28 (Low)

📘 Bologna— turkey ☞ 28 (Low)

📘 Bratwurst, cooked ☞ 28 (Low)

📘 Broccoli cheese soup—prepared with milk ☞ 27 (Low)

📘 Broccoli soup ☞ 27 (Low)

📘 Burger—beef, with tomato, onion, ketchup, mixed lettuce, and cheese, with hamburger bun (small) ☞ 63 (Medium)

📘 Burger—Fillet-O-Fish, fish patty, tartare sauce and cheese on a burger bun ☞ 66 (Medium)

📘 Burger—Lean beef patty, tomato, onion, mixed lettuce, cheese, and burger sauce on a burger bun ☞ 66 (Medium)

📘 Burger—vegetarian, with tomato, onion, veggie burger, mixed lettuce, and vegan alternative cheese, with hamburger bun (small) ☞ 59 (Low)

📘 Burrito—beef, with beans, sour cream and cheese ☞ 33 (Low)

📘 Burrito—sausage, cheese, eggs and vegetables ☞ 31 (Low)

📘 Burrito—with beef and beans ☞ 34 (Low)

📘 Burrito—with beef and cheese, whitout beans ☞ 30 (Low)

- Burrito—with beef, with beans, and cheese ☛ 34 (Low)
- Burrito—with cheese, beans, without meat or poultry ☛ 34 (Low)
- Canadian bacon, cooked ☛ 50 (Low)
- Carrot soup—prepared with milk ☛ 37 (Low)
- Cauliflower soup—prepared with milk ☛ 27 (Low)
- Celery soup—made with milk or water, average value ☛ 27 (Low)
- Celery soup—prepared with milk ☛ 27 (Low)
- Celery soup—prepared with water ☛ 27 (Low)
- Cheddar cheese soup ☛ 27 (Low)
- Chicken and Beef sausage— smoked ☛ 28 (Low)
- Chicken and mushroom soup—prepared with milk ☛ 27 (Low)
- Chicken and noodles—no sauce ☛ 40 (Low)
- Chicken and noodles—with cream or white sauce ☛ 46 (Low)
- Chicken fillet sandwich—broiled, cheese, lettuce, tomato, spread, and bun ☛ 59 (Medium)
- Chicken fillet sandwich—broiled, lettuce, tomato, spread and whole-wheat roll ☛ 69 (Medium)
- Chicken garden salad—tomato, carrots, other vegetables, no potato, no dressing ☛ 32 (Low)
- Chicken gumbo soup ☛ 38 (Low)
- Chicken korma made with rice ☛ 45 (Low)
- Chicken Nuggets—eaten with sweet Thai Chili sauce ☛ 64 (Medium)
- Chicken nuggets—frozen, reheated ☛ 56 (Medium)
- Chicken or turkey—cacciatore ☛ 61 (Medium)

- Chicken patty sandwich ☞ 67 (Medium)
- Chicken Pomodoro—reheated, convenience meal ☞ 46 (Low)
- Chicken salad ☞ 41 (Low)
- Chicken teriyaki ☞ 57 (Medium)
- Chicken with barbecue sauce ☞ 38 (Low)
- Chicken with vegetables—carrots, broccoli, dark-green leafy without sauce ☞ 43 (Low)
- Chicken with vegetables—carrots, broccoli, dark-green leafy, with soy-based sauce ☞ 55 (Low)
- Chicken—Indian Chicken Tikka Masala ☞ 46 (Low)
- Chicken—Indian Style Butter with Rice: $Gi \cong 43$
- Chilaquiles—prepared with corn tortilla, tomato, sauce, cheese, boiled and pinto beans ☞ 51 (Low)
- Chiles rellenos ☞ 35 (Low)
- Chili beef noodles ☞ 42 (Low)
- Chili con carne—beans ☞ 34 (Low)
- Chili con carne—beans and cheese ☞ 34 (Low)
- Chili con carne—beans and rice ☞ 55 (Low)
- Chili con carne—beans, macaroni ☞ 41 (Low)
- Chili con carne—beans, made with chicken ☞ 34 (Low)
- Chili con carne—beans, made with turkey ☞ 34 (Low)
- Chili con carne—beans, made with venison/deer ☞ 34 (Low)
- Chili con carne—beans, prepared with pork ☞ 34 (Low)
- Chili con carne—made from navy beans ☞ 34 (Low)

- 📕 Chili con carne—without beans ☛ 37 (Low)
- 📕 Chorizos ☛ 28 (Low)
- 📕 Chorizos ☛ 28 (Low)
- 📕 Chow mein chicken ☛ 55 (Low)
- 📕 Classic French baguette with 10 g butter and two slices of ham ☛ 59 (Medium)
- 📕 Cold cut—Average Value ☛ 28 (Low)
- 📕 Cottage pie ☛ 65 (Medium)
- 📕 Cumberland fish pie ☛ 40 (Low)
- 📕 Cumberland pie ☛ 29 (Low)
- 📕 Deer bologna ☛ 28 (Low)
- 📕 Egg tart ☛ 45 (Low)
- 📕 Fajita with chicken and vegetables ☛ 31 (Low)
- 📕 Fajitas with chicken ☛ 42 (Low)
- 📕 Fajitas with turkey ☛ 42 (Low)
- 📕 Fish fingers ☛ 48 (Low)
- 📕 Frankfurter, Wiener, or Hot Dog—beef ☛ 28 (Low)
- 📕 Frankfurter, Wiener, or Hot Dog—beef and pork ☛ 28 (Low)
- 📕 Frankfurter, Wiener, or Hot Dog—beef and pork, low-fat ☛ 28 (Low)
- 📕 Frankfurter, Wiener, or Hot Dog—beef, low-fat ☛ 28 (Low)
- 📕 Frankfurter, Wiener, or Hot Dog—chicken ☛ 28 (Low)
- 📕 Frankfurter, Wiener, or Hot Dog—low salt ☛ 28 (Low)
- 📕 Frankfurter, Wiener, or Hot Dog—meat & poultry, low-fat ☛

THE ESSENTIAL FOODS LISTS FOR THE GLYCEMIC INDEX DIET

28 (Low)

📕 Frankfurter, Wiener, or Hot Dog—meat and poultry ☛ 28 (Low)

📕 Frankfurter, Wiener, or Hot Dog—meat and poultry, fat free ☛ 28 (Low)

📕 Frankfurter, Wiener, or Hot Dog—turkey ☛ 28 (Low)

📕 Frankfurter, wiener, or hot dog, Average Value ☛ 28 (Low)

📕 Fruit salad— with citrus fruits ☛ 41 (Low)

📕 Fruit salad—no citrus fruits with cream substitute ☛ 46 (Low)

📕 Fruit salad—with cream, no citrus fruits ☛ 48 (Low)

📕 Fruit salad—with mayonnaise ☛ 49 (Low)

📕 Fruit—chocolate covered ☛ 54 (Low)

📕 Italian pie, without meat or poultry ☛ 60 (Medium)

📕 Knockwurst ☛ 28 (Low)

📕 Lasagna—beef ☛ 47 (Low)

📕 Lasagna—meat ☛ 47 (Low)

📕 Lasagna—type not specified ☛ 47 (Low)

📕 Lasagna—vegetarian, no potato ☛ 36 (Low)

📕 Luncheon loaf—with olive, pickle, and/or pimiento ☛ 28 (Low)

📕 Luncheon meat— Average Value ☛ 28 (Low)

📕 Macaroni—creamed, with cheese ☛ 43 (Low)

📕 Macaroni—salad ☛ 45 (Low)

📕 Meatloaf—prepared with beef ☛ 61 (Medium)

📕 Meatloaf—prepared with beef, tomato sauce ☛ 56 (Medium)

📕 Meatloaf—prepared with chicken or turkey ☛ 60 (Medium)

📖 Mettwurst ☛ 28 (Low)

📖 Mixed vegetables—from canned, corn, carrots, lima beans, peas, and green beans, cooked, without fat ☛ 43 (Low)

📖 Mixed vegetables—from corn, carrots, lima beans, peas, and green beans, without fat ☛ 43 (Low)

📖 Mixed vegetables—from frozen, corn, lima beans, carrots, peas, and green beans, without fat ☛ 43 (Low)

📖 Mortadella ☛ 28 (Low)

📖 Pasta salad ☛ 46 (Low)

📖 Pepper steak ☛ 46 (Low)

📖 Pepperoni ☛ 28 (Low)

📖 Pizza—cheese, Not Specified as to the type of crust ☛ 60 (Medium)

📖 Pizza—cheese, thick-crust ☛ 60 (Medium)

📖 Pizza—cheese, thin-crust ☛ 60 (Medium)

📖 Pizza—cheese, with fruit, thick crust ☛ 60 (Medium)

📖 Pizza—cheese, with vegetables, Not Specified as to the type of crust ☛ 49 (Low)

📖 Pizza—cheese, with vegetables, thick crust ☛ 49 (Low)

📖 Pizza—cheese, with vegetables, thin-crust ☛ 49 (Low)

📖 Pizza—with meat and fruit, thick crust ☛ 36 (Low)

📖 Pizza—with meat and fruit, thin-crust ☛ 30 (Low)

📖 Pizza—with meat and vegetables, low-fat, thin-crust ☛ 30 (Low)

📖 Pizza—with meat and vegetables, Not Specified as to the type of crust ☛ 30 (Low)

THE ESSENTIAL FOODS LISTS FOR THE GLYCEMIC INDEX DIET

- Pizza—with meat and vegetables, thick crust — 36 (Low)
- Pizza—with meat and vegetables, thin-crust — 30 (Low)
- Pizza—with meat, Not Specified as to the type of crust — 30 (Low)
- Pizza—with meat, thick crust — 36 (Low)
- Pizza—with meat, thin-crust — 30 (Low)
- Polish sausage — 28 (Low)
- Pork roll—cured, fried — 28 (Low)
- Potato salad — 66 (Medium)
- Potato salad—German-style — 68 (Medium)
- Potato salad—with egg — 66 (Medium)
- Pudding—bread — 62 (Medium)
- Pudding—fruit, vanilla wafers — 59 (Medium)
- Roast beef sandwich—with cheese — 69 (Medium)
- Salami—Average Value — 28 (Low)
- Salami—beef — 28 (Low)
- Salami—dry or hard — 28 (Low)
- Salami—soft, cooked — 28 (Low)
- Salisbury steak with gravy — 64 (Medium)
- Sandwich loaf—luncheon meat — 28 (Low)
- Sausage— low-fat, smoked, turkey, pork, and beef — 28 (Low)
- Sausage—Average Value — 28 (Low)
- Sausage—from fresh, cooked bulk, patty or link, with turkey and pork — 28 (Low)
- Sausage—from fresh, pork, bulk, patty or link, cooked — 28 (Low)

- Sausage—from fresh, pork, country style, cooked 🐖 28 (Low)
- Sausage—Italian 🐖 28 (Low)
- Sausage—Pork and Beef 🐖 28 (Low)
- Sausage—Pork and Beef brown and serve, cooked 🐖 28 (Low)
- Sausage—pork, brown and serve, cooked 🐖 28 (Low)
- Sausage—reduced fat, smoked, turkey, pork, and beef 🐖 28 (Low)
- Sausage—Smoked link , pork 🐖 28 (Low)
- Sausage—Smoked link, pork and beef 🐖 28 (Low)
- Sausage—smoked, pork 🐖 28 (Low)
- Sausage—smoked, turkey 🐖 28 (Low)
- Sausage—Vienna, canned 🐖 28 (Low)
- Sausage—Vienna, canned, chicken 🐖 28 (Low)
- Scrapple—cooked 🐖 28 (Low)
- Soft taco with beef 🐖 30 (Low)
- Souse 🐖 28 (Low)
- Spaghetti bolognaise—home recipe 🐖 52 (Low)
- Stuffed bun—meat, shallots, steamed 🐖 39 (Low)
- Sushi—average 🐖 55 (Low)
- Sushi—roasted sea algae, vinegar and rice 🐖 55 (Low)
- Sushi, salmon 🐖 55 (Low)
- Sweet and sour turkey 🐖 53 (Low)
- Taco salad—with beef, cheese, corn chips 🐖 56 (Medium)
- Taco—with beans, meat, lettuce, cheese, tomato and salsa 🐖 55 (Low)

THE ESSENTIAL FOODS LISTS FOR THE GLYCEMIC INDEX DIET

- Taco—with beef, lettuce and cheese ☞ 68 (Medium)
- Taco—with beef, tomato, lettuce, cheese, and salsa ☞ 58 (Medium)
- Tamale prepared with meat and/or chicken ☞ 62 (Medium)
- Thuringer ☞ 28 (Low)
- Tomato and Herb Chicken ☞ 52 (Low)
- Tuna fish sandwich ☞ 46 (Low)
- Turkey and pork sausage ☞ 28 (Low)
- Turkey bacon—cooked ☞ 50 (Low)
- Turkey bacon—cooked ☞ 50 (Low)
- Turkey salad ☞ 41 (Low)
- Turkey sausage—smoked ☞ 28 (Low)
- Turkey teriyaki ☞ 57 (Medium)
- Turkey with barbecue sauce ☞ 38 (Low)
- Turkey, pork, and beef sausage—low-fat, smoked ☞ 28 (Low)

20

SOUPS: LOW AND MEDIUM GLYCEMIC INDEX FOODS

- Asparagus soup—made with milk or water ☛ 27 (Low)
- Asparagus soup—prepared with milk ☛ 27 (Low)
- Barley soup ☛ 25 (Low)
- Bean and ham soup—chunky style ☛ 64 (Medium)
- Bean and ham soup—home recipe ☛ 64 (Medium)
- Bean and rice soup ☛ 42.2 (Low)
- Bean soup—average ☛ 64 (Medium)
- Bean soup—home recipe ☛ 64 (Medium)
- Bean soup—mixed beans ☛ 64 (Medium)
- Bean soup—with bacon or pork ☛ 64 (Medium)
- Bean soup—with macaroni ☛ 37.8 (Low)
- Bean soup—with macaroni and meat ☛ 38.3 (Low)
- Bean soup—with vegetables and rice ☛ 55.3 (Medium)

THE ESSENTIAL FOODS LISTS FOR THE GLYCEMIC INDEX DIET

- Beef and rice noodle soup ☛ 53 (Low)
- Beef noodle soup ☛ 42 (Low)
- Beef noodle soup—home recipe ☛ 42 (Low)
- Beef noodle soup—Sopa de carne y fideos ☛ 42 (Low)
- Beef pot pie ☛ 45 (Low)
- Beef rice soup ☛ 64 (Low)
- Beef stroganoff soup—chunky style ☛ 42 (Low)
- Beef stroganoff—with noodles ☛ 46 (Low)
- Beef vegetable soup—Sopa caldo de Res ☛ 38 (Low)
- Beef vegetable soup—with noodles, stew type, chunky style ☛ 40 (Low)
- Beef vegetable soup—with potato, stew type ☛ 44 (Low)
- Beef vegetable soup—with rice, stew type, chunky style ☛ 51 (Low)
- Beef, rice, and vegetables soup —not carrots, not broccoli ☛ 49.1 (Low)
- Beef, rice, and vegetables soup—with carrots, broccoli ☛ 47.4 (Low)
- Black bean soup ☛ 64 (Medium)
- Broccoli cheese soup—prepared with milk ☛ 27 (Low)
- Broccoli soup ☛ 27 (Low)
- Carrot soup—prepared with milk ☛ 37 (Low)
- Cauliflower soup—prepared with milk ☛ 27 (Low)
- Celery soup—made with milk or water, average value ☛ 27 (Low)
- Celery soup—prepared with milk ☛ 27 (Low)

- Celery soup—prepared with water ☞ 27 (Low)
- Cheddar cheese soup ☞ 27 (Low)
- Chicken and mushroom soup—prepared with milk ☞ 27 (Low)
- Chicken gumbo soup ☞ 38 (Low)
- Chicken noodle soup ☞ 42 (Low)
- Chicken noodle soup—canned ☞ 42 (Low)
- Chicken noodle soup—canned ☞ 42 (Low)
- Chicken noodle soup—chunky style ☞ 40 (Low)
- Chicken noodle soup—cream of ☞ 34.5 (Low)
- Chicken noodle soup—home recipe ☞ 42 (Low)
- Chicken or turkey rice soup—home recipe ☞ 64 (Medium)
- Chicken or turkey soup—canned, prepared with milk ☞ 27 (Low)
- Chicken or turkey soup—canned, prepared with water ☞ 27 (Low)
- Chicken or turkey soup—canned, undiluted ☞ 27 (Low)
- Chicken or turkey soup—prepared with milk ☞ 27 (Low)
- Chicken or turkey soup—prepared with water ☞ 27 (Low)
- Chicken or turkey soup—with milk or water, average value ☞ 27 (Low)
- Chicken or turkey vegetable soup—home recipe ☞ 38 (Low)
- Chicken or turkey vegetable soup—stew type ☞ 38 (Low)
- Chicken rice soup ☞ 64 (Medium)
- Chicken rice soup—canned ☞ 64 (Medium)
- Chicken rice soup—Sopa de pollo con arroz ☞ 64 (Medium)
- Chicken soup ☞ 42 (Low)

THE ESSENTIAL FOODS LISTS FOR THE GLYCEMIC INDEX DIET

- Chicken soup—with noodles and potatoes ☛ 57 (Medium)
- Chicken soup—with vegetables, Oriental style ☛ 38 (Low)
- Chicken vegetable soup—with noodles, chunky style ☛ 40 (Low)
- Chicken vegetable soup—with potato, cheese, chunky style ☛ 44 (Low)
- Chicken vegetable soup—with rice, stew type ☛ 51 (Low)
- Chickpea soup ☛ 64 (Low)
- Chili beef soup ☛ 51 (Low)
- Chili beef soup—chunky style ☛ 51 (Low)
- Corn soup—prepared with milk ☛ 40.5 (Low)
- Corn soup—prepared with water ☛ 40.5 (Low)
- Crab soup—prepared with milk ☛ 27 (Low)
- Crab soup—tomato-base ☛ 38 (Low)
- Cucumber soup—prepared with milk ☛ 27 (Low)
- Dark-green leafy vegetable soup ☛ 38 (Low)
- Dark-green leafy vegetable soup, meatless ☛ 38 (Low)
- Ham soup— with chunky pea ☛ 66 (Medium)
- Ham, potato, and rice soup ☛ 51 (Low)
- Instant soup rice ☛ 64 (Low)
- Instant soup, noodle ☛ 42 (Low)
- Instant soup, noodle—with chicken, egg, or shrimp ☛ 42 (Low)
- Leek soup—prepared with milk ☛ 27 (Low)
- Lentil soup ☛ 44 (Low)
- Lima bean soup ☛ 60 (Medium)

- Macaroni and potato soup ☛ 62.5 (Medium)
- Meat and corn hominy soup ☛ 40 (Low)
- Meatball soup—Sopa de Albondigas ☛ 38 (Low)
- Minestrone soup—canned ☛ 39 (Low)
- Minestrone soup—home recipe ☛ 39 (Low)
- Mushroom soup—average value ☛ 27 (Low)
- Mushroom soup—canned, made with milk, ☛ 27 (Low)
- Mushroom soup—cream of, with milk ☛ 27 (Low)
- Mushroom soup—made with water, cream of ☛ 27 (Low)
- Mushroom soup—prepared with water ☛ 27 (Low)
- Mushroom soup—undiluted ☛ 27 (Low)
- Noodle and potato soup ☛ 42 (Low)
- Noodle soup with vegetable—Oriental style ☛ 40 (Low)
- Noodle soup—average value ☛ 42 (Low)
- Noodle soup—with fish ball, and/or shrimp, and dark green leafy vegetable ☛ 42 (Low)
- Oxtail soup ☛ 38 (Low)
- Pasta salad—macaroni or noodles, and vegetables ☛ 45.6 (Low)
- Pasta—canned, with tomato sauce and cheese ☛ 40 (Low)
- Pasta—canned, with tomato sauce and meatballs ☛ 52 (Low)
- Pasta—with carbonara sauce ☛ 42 (Low)
- Pasta—with cheese and meat sauce ☛ 52 (Low)
- Pasta—with meat sauce ☛ 52 (Low)

- Pasta—without meat or poultry, with cheese and tomato sauce ☞ 40 (Low)
- Pasta—without meat or poultry, with tomato sauce ☞ 40 (Low)
- Pea soup—canned, made with water ☞ 66 (Medium)
- Pea soup—common ☞ 66 (Medium)
- Pea soup—instant type ☞ 66 (Medium)
- Pea soup—made with mill ☞ 46.5 (Low)
- Pea soup—made with water ☞ 66 (Medium)
- Pork and rice soup—stew type / chunky style ☞ 51 (Low)
- Pork vegetable soup—with noodles, stew type /chunky style ☞ 40 (Low)
- Pork with vegetable soup—no carrots, no dark-green leafy ☞ 38 (Low)
- Pork, vegetable soup—with potatoes /stew type ☞ 38 (Low)
- Potato and cheese soup ☞ 53.9 (Low)
- Potato soup— prepared with milk ☞ 49.5 (Low)
- Potato soup—average value ☞ 49.5 (Low)
- Potato soup—made with water ☞ 49.5 (Low)
- Rice and potato soup—Puerto Rican style ☞ 64 (Medium)
- Rice soup—average value ☞ 64 (Medium)
- Salmon soup—cream style ☞ 27 (Low)
- Seasoned shredded soup with meat ☞ 50 (Low)
- Shrimp soup—prepared with milk ☞ 27 (Low)
- Soup—average value ☞ 38 (Low)

DR. H. MAHER

- Soup—mostly noodles ☛ 42 (Low)
- Soybean soup—made with milk ☛ 43.5 (Low)
- Soybean soup—miso broth ☛ 29.2 (Low)
- Spaghetti—cooked, average value ☛ 42 (Low)
- Spaghetti—cooked, with fat ☛ 42 (Low)
- Spaghetti—whole wheat spaghetti, with tomato sauce and meat ☛ 52 (Low)
- Spaghetti—with clam sauce ☛ 40 (Low)
- Spaghetti—with red clam sauce ☛ 40 (Low)
- Spaghetti—with tomato sauce and hot dogs ☛ 52 (Low)
- Spaghetti—with tomato sauce and meatballs ☛ 52 (Low)
- Spaghetti—with tomato sauce and poultry ☛ 52 (Low)
- Spaghetti—with white clam sauce ☛ 42 (Low)
- Spaghetti—without meat or poultry, tomato sauce ☛ 40 (Low)
- Spaghetti,—cooked, whitout fat ☛ 42 (Low)
- Split pea soup ☛ 60 (Medium)
- Split pea soup—canned ☛ 60 (Medium)
- Split peas soup—with ham ☛ 60 (Medium)
- Split peas soup—with ham, canned ☛ 60 (Medium)
- Tomato beef noodle soup—made with water ☛ 40 (Low)
- Tomato beef soup—made with water ☛ 38 (Low)
- Tomato noodle soup—made with water ☛ 40 (Low)
- Tomato soup—average value ☛ 38 (Low)
- Tomato soup—canned ☛ 38 (Low)

- Tomato soup—canned, undiluted — 38 (Low)
- Tomato soup—instant type, made with water — 38 (Low)
- Tomato soup—made with water — 38 (Low)
- Tomato soup—prepared with milk — 35.7 (Low)
- Tomato vegetable soup—made with water — 38 (Low)
- Tomato vegetable soup—with noodles, made with water — 40 (Low)
- Turkey noodle soup — 42 (Low)
- Turkey noodle soup—home recipe — 42 (Low)
- Vegetable bean soup—ready-to-serve or prepared with water — 39 (Low)
- Vegetable beef soup with rice—home recipe — 51 (Low)
- Vegetable beef soup with rice—ready-to-serve or prepared with water — 51 (Low)
- Vegetable beef soup—canned, undiluted — 38 (Low)
- Vegetable beef soup—chunky style — 38 (Low)
- Vegetable beef soup—home recipe — 38 (Low)
- Vegetable beef soup—home recipe, with noodles or pasta — 40 (Low)
- Vegetable beef soup—prepared with water — 38 (Low)
- Vegetable chicken noodle soup—prepared with water — 40 (Low)
- Vegetable chicken or turkey soup—made with water — 38 (Low)
- Vegetable chicken rice soup—with water or ready-to-serve — 51 (Low)
- Vegetable chicken soup—canned, prepared with water — 38 (Low)

- Vegetable noodle soup—canned, water or ready-to-serve ☞ 40 (Low)
- Vegetable noodle soup—home recipe ☞ 40 (Low)
- Vegetable noodle soup—with water ☞ 40 (Low)
- Vegetable rice soup—prepared with water ☞ 51 (Low)
- Vegetable soup—canned, low sodium, water ☞ 38 (Low)
- Vegetable soup—canned, undiluted ☞ 38 (Low)
- Vegetable soup—chunky style ☞ 38 (Low)
- Vegetable soup—home recipe ☞ 38 (Low)
- Vegetable soup—made from dry mix ☞ 38 (Low)
- Vegetable soup—made with water or ready-to-serve ☞ 38 (Low)
- Vegetable soup—prepared with dry mix, low sodium, water ☞ 32.5 (Low)
- Vegetable soup—prepared with milk ☞ 32.5 (Low)
- Vegetable soup—with chicken broth ☞ 38 (Low)
- Vegetable soup—with pasta, chunky style ☞ 40 (Low)
- Vegetarian vegetable soup—made with water ☞ 38 (Low)
- Zucchini soup—made with milk ☞ 27 (Low)

21

SAUCES, OILS AND SALAD DRESSING: LOW AND MEDIUM GLYCEMIC INDEX FOODS

- Sauce—Alfredo ☛ 27 (Low)
- Beef Tallow ☛ 0 (Low)
- Clarified Butter ☛ 0 (Low)
- Cocktail sauce ☛ 38 (Low)
- Dressing—Blue or roquefort ☛ 50 (Low)
- Dressing—Blue or roquefort, low-calorie ☛ 50 (Low)
- Dressing—Blue or roquefort, reduced calorie ☛ 50 (Low)
- Dressing—Blue or roquefort, reduced calorie, fat-free ☛ 50 (Low)
- Dressing—Caesar ☛ 50 (Low)
- Dressing—Caesar, low-calorie ☛ 50 (Low)
- Dressing—Coleslaw ☛ 50 (Low)
- Dressing—Coleslaw, reduced calorie ☛ 50 (Low)
- Dressing—Cream cheese ☛ 50 (Low)

- Dressing—Creamy, prepared with sour cream, buttermilk and oil ☞ 50 (Low)

- Dressing—Creamy, prepared with sour cream, diet ☞ 50 (Low)

- Dressing—Creamy, prepared with sour cream, low calorie, cholesterol free ☞ 50 (Low)

- Dressing—Creamy, prepared with sour cream, or buttermilk and oil ☞ 50 (Low)

- Dressing—Creamy, prepared with sour cream, reduced calorie ☞ 50 (Low)

- Dressing—Creamy, prepared with sour cream, reduced calorie, cholesterol-free ☞ 50 (Low)

- Dressing—Feta Cheese ☞ 50 (Low)

- Dressing—French ☞ 50 (Low)

- Dressing—French, low calorie, fat free ☞ 50 (Low)

- Dressing—French, reduced calorie ☞ 50 (Low)

- Dressing—Green Goddess ☞ 50 (Low)

- Dressing—Honey mustard ☞ 50 (Low)

- Dressing—Italian dressing ☞ 50 (Low)

- Dressing—Italian, diet or reduced calorie ☞ 50 (Low)

- Dressing—Italian, diet or reduced calorie, fat free ☞ 50 (Low)

- Dressing—Italian, reduced calorie ☞ 50 (Low)

- Dressing—Korean ☞ 50 (Low)

- Dressing—Mayonnaise-type salad, cholesterol-free ☞ 50 (Low)

- Dressing—Mayonnaise-type salad, diet ☞ 50 (Low)

- Dressing—Mayonnaise-type salad, fat-free ☞ 50 (Low)

- Dressing—Mayonnaise-type salad, low calorie ☞ 50 (Low)
- Dressing—Mayonnaise-type salad, Regular ☞ 50 (Low)
- Dressing—Milk, vinegar based ☞ 50 (Low)
- Dressing—Peppercorn ☞ 50 (Low)
- Dressing—Poppy seed ☞ 50 (Low)
- Dressing—Rice ☞ 64 (Low)
- Dressing—Russian ☞ 50 (Low)
- Dressing—Russian, low calorie ☞ 50 (Low)
- Dressing—Salad dressing, low-calorie, without oil ☞ 50 (Low)
- Dressing—Salad, common ☞ 50 (Low)
- Dressing—Salad, low calorie ☞ 50 (Low)
- Dressing—Sesame ☞ 50 (Low)
- Dressing—Sweet and sour ☞ 50 (Low)
- Dressing—Thousand Island Regular ☞ 50 (Low)
- Dressing—Thousand Island, low-calorie ☞ 50 (Low)
- Dressing—Thousand Island, reduced calorie, cholesterol free ☞ 50 (Low)
- Dressing—Vinegar based ☞ 50 (Low)
- Dressing—Yogurt ☞ 50 (Low)
- Duck Fat ☞ 0 (Low)
- French dressing, low-calorie ☞ 50 (Low)
- Gravy—giblet ☞ 50 (Low)
- Gravy—meat or poultry, with wine ☞ 50 (Low)
- Gravy—meat, with fruit ☞ 50 (Low)

- Gravy—mushroom ☞ 50 (Low)
- Gravy—poultry ☞ 38 (Low)
- Gravy—poultry, with wine ☞ 50 (Low)
- Margarine ☞ 0 (Low)
- Mayonnaise—diet or low-calorie ☞ 50 (Low)
- Mayonnaise—diet or low-calorie, low sodium ☞ 50 (Low)
- Mayonnaise—imitation ☞ 50 (Low)
- Mayonnaise—low caloriet, cholesterol-free ☞ 50 (Low)
- Mayonnaise—made with tofu ☞ 50 (Low)
- Mayonnaise—made with yogurt ☞ 50 (Low)
- Mayonnaise, regular ☞ 50 (Low)
- Mustard greens—from canned, cooked, average value ☞ 32 (Low)
- Mustard greens—from canned, cooked, with fat ☞ 32 (Low)
- Mustard greens—from canned, cooked, without fat ☞ 32 (Low)
- Mustard greens—from fresh, cooked, with fat ☞ 32 (Low)
- Mustard greens—from fresh, cooked, without fat ☞ 32 (Low)
- Mustard greens—from frozen, cooked, average value ☞ 32 (Low)
- Mustard greens—from frozen, cooked, with fat ☞ 32 (Low)
- Mustard greens—from frozen, cooked, without fat ☞ 32 (Low)
- Mustard pickles ☞ 32 (Low)
- Oil—Avocado ☞ 0 (Low)
- Oil—Canola ☞ 0 (Low)
- Oil—Coconut ☞ 0 (Low)

THE ESSENTIAL FOODS LISTS FOR THE GLYCEMIC INDEX DIET

- Oil—Corn ☞ 0 (Low)
- Oil—Extra-virgin olive ☞ 0 (Low)
- Oil—Flaxseed ☞ 0 (Low)
- Oil—Grapeseed ☞ 0 (Low)
- Oil—Hazelnut ☞ 0 (Low)
- Oil—Hemp seed ☞ 0 (Low)
- Oil—Macadamia Nut ☞ 0 (Low)
- Oil—Olive ☞ 0 (Low)
- Oil—Palm ☞ 0 (Low)
- Oil—Peanut ☞ 0 (Low)
- Oil—Rice Bran ☞ 0 (Low)
- Oil—Sesame ☞ 0 (Low)
- Oil—Sunflower ☞ 0 (Low)
- Oil—Vegetable ☞ 0 (Low)
- Oil—Walnut ☞ 32 (Low)
- Sauce—Cheese ☞ 27 (Low)
- Sauce—Cheese prepared with lowfat cheese ☞ 27 (Low)
- Sauce—Clam, white ☞ 27 (Low)
- Sauce—Tomato ☞ 38 (Low)
- Sauce—Tomato chili ☞ 38 (Low)
- Sauce—Tomato, low sodium ☞ 27 (Low)
- Sauce—White, or milk sauce ☞ 50 (Low)
- Spaghetti sauce ☞ 38 (Low)

- Spaghetti sauce—canned, with meat, canned ☞ 38 (Low)
- Spaghetti sauce—homemade, fat free ☞ 38 (Low)
- Spaghetti sauce—homemade, low salt ☞ 38 (Low)
- Spaghetti sauce—homemade, with beef ☞ 38 (Low)
- Spaghetti sauce—homemade, with combination of meats ☞ 38 (Low)
- Spaghetti sauce—homemade, with lamb ☞ 38 (Low)
- Spaghetti sauce—homemade, with meat ☞ 38 (Low)
- Spaghetti sauce—homemade, with poultry ☞ 38 (Low)
- Vinegar, sugar, and water dressing ☞ 0 (Low)

22
SPICES AND HERBS: LOW AND MEDIUM GLYCEMIC INDEX FOODS

- Allspice ► 15 (Low)
- Anise seeds ► 0.0 (Low)
- Asian chives ► 15 (Low)
- Bay leaves ► 23 (Low)
- Black cumin ► 0.0 (Low)
- Black pepper ► 44 (Low)
- capers ► 20 (Low)
- Caraway ► 5 (Low)
- Cayenne pepper ► 32 (Low)
- Celery seed ► 32 (Low)
- Chiles ► 42 (Low)
- chilli ► 15 (Low)
- Chives ► 15 (Low)

- Cilantro ☛ 32 (Low)
- Coriander seed ☛ 33 (Low)
- Coriander seeds ☛ 33 (Low)
- Cumin ☛ 0.0 (Low)
- Curry Leaves ☛ 5 (Low)
- Curry powder ☛ 5 (Low)
- curry powder ☛ 5 (Low)
- Dill seed ☛ 15 (Low)
- Fennel seeds ☛ 16 (Low)
- Fenugreek ☛ 25 (Low)
- Fenugreek Leaves ☛ 25 (Low)
- Five Spice Powder ☛ Low
- Garlic chives ☛ 15 (Low)
- Lemon Balm ☛ 15 (Low)
- Lemongrass ☛ 45 (Low)
- Lime Leaves ☛ 32 (Low)
- Mint ☛ 10 (Low)
- Mustard Seed ☛ 32 (Low)
- Nutmeg ☛ 46 (Low)
- Oregano ☛ 5 (Low)
- Paprika ☛ 15 (Low)
- Parsley ☛ 32 (Low)
- poppy seeds ☛ 5 (Low)

THE ESSENTIAL FOODS LISTS FOR THE GLYCEMIC INDEX DIET

- Sage ☞ 15 (Low)
- Savory ☞ 16 (Low)
- Sesame seeds ☞ 31 (Low)
- Sumac ☞ 43 (Low)
- Summer Savoy ☞ 21 (Low)
- tarragon ☞ 15 (Low)
- Thyme ☞ 51 (Low)
- Turmeric ☞ 15 (Low)
- Vanilla ☞ 16 (Low)
- wasabi powder ☞ 31 (Low)
- Watercress ☞ 32 (Low)
- Wild garlic ☞ 11 (Low)

23
VEGETABLES: LOW AND MEDIUM GLYCEMIC INDEX FOODS

- Alfalfa sprouts, raw ➤ 32 (Low)
- Algae, dried ➤ 32 (Low)
- Apple, pickled ➤ 38 (Low)
- Artichoke— globe (French), cooked, from canned ➤ 32 (Low)
- Artichoke— globe (French), cooked, from fresh ➤ 32 (Low)
- Artichoke— globe (French), cooked, from fresh, with fat ➤ 32 (Low)
- Artichoke— globe (French), cooked, from fresh, without fat ➤ 32 (Low)
- Artichoke— globe (French), cooked, from frozen, Not Specified as to with fat ➤ 32 (Low)
- Artichoke— globe (French), cooked, (average value) ➤ 32 (Low)
- Artichoke— globe (French), cooked, (average value), without fat ➤ 32 (Low)
- Artichoke— Jerusalem, raw ➤ 32 (Low)

THE ESSENTIAL FOODS LISTS FOR THE GLYCEMIC INDEX DIET

- Artichoke— salad in oil ☛ 32 (Low)
- Asparagus— cooked, from canned, Not Specified as to with fat ☛ 32 (Low)
- Asparagus— cooked, from canned, with fat ☛ 32 (Low)
- Asparagus— cooked, from canned, without fat ☛ 32 (Low)
- Asparagus— cooked, from fresh, Not Specified as to with fat ☛ 32 (Low)
- Asparagus— cooked, from fresh, with fat ☛ 32 (Low)
- Asparagus— cooked, from fresh, without fat ☛ 32 (Low)
- Asparagus— cooked, from frozen, with fat ☛ 32 (Low)
- Asparagus— cooked, from frozen, without fat ☛ 32 (Low)
- Asparagus— cooked, Not Specified as to form, Not Specified as to with fat ☛ 32 (Low)
- Asparagus— cooked, Not Specified as to form, with fat ☛ 32 (Low)
- Asparagus— cooked, Not Specified as to form, without fat ☛ 32 (Low)
- Asparagus— from canned, creamed or with cheese sauce ☛ 28 (Low)
- Asparagus— from fresh, creamed or with cheese sauce ☛ 29 (Low)
- Asparagus— raw ☛ 32 (Low)
- Bamboo shoots—cooked, with fat ☛ 32 (Low)
- Bamboo shoots—cooked, without fat ☛ 32 (Low)
- Bean sprouts— cooked, from canned, with fat ☛ 32 (Low)
- Bean sprouts— cooked, from canned, without fat ☛ 32 (Low)

- Bean sprouts— cooked, from fresh, Not Specified as to with fat ☛ 32 (Low)

- Bean sprouts— cooked, from fresh, with fat ☛ 32 (Low)

- Bean sprouts— cooked, from fresh, without fat ☛ 32 (Low)

- Bean sprouts— cooked, Not Specified as to form, Not Specified as to with fat ☛ 32 (Low)

- Bean sprouts— cooked, Not Specified as to form, with fat ☛ 32 (Low)

- Bean sprouts— raw (soybean or mung) ☛ 32 (Low)

- Beans, green string—with tomatoes, cooked, without fat ☛ 35 (Low)

- Beans, green—with pinto beans, cooked, without fat ☛ 38 (Low)

- Beet greens—raw ☛ 32 (Low)

- Bitter melon—cooked, without fat ☛ 32 (Low)

- Broccoflower—cooked, without fat ☛ 32 (Low)

- Broccoli—cooked, from fresh, without fat ☛ 32 (Low)

- Broccoli—cooked, from frozen, without fat ☛ 32 (Low)

- Broccoli—cooked, Not Specified as to form, without fat ☛ 32 (Low)

- Broccoli—raw ☛ 32 (Low)

- Brussels sprouts—cooked, from fresh, without fat ☛ 32 (Low)

- Brussels sprouts—cooked, from frozen, without fat ☛ 32 (Low)

- Brussels sprouts—cooked, Not Specified as to form, without fat ☛ 32 (Low)

- Brussels sprouts—raw ☛ 32 (Low)

THE ESSENTIAL FOODS LISTS FOR THE GLYCEMIC INDEX DIET

- Cabbage—Chinese, cooked, Not Specified as to with fat ► 32 (Low)
- Cabbage—Chinese, cooked, with fat ► 32 (Low)
- Cabbage—Chinese, cooked, without fat ► 32 (Low)
- Cabbage—Chinese, raw ► 32 (Low)
- Cabbage—Chinese, salad, with dressing ► 32 (Low)
- Cabbage—fresh, pickled, Japanese style ► 32 (Low)
- Cabbage—green, cooked, Not Specified as to with fat ► 32 (Low)
- Cabbage—green, cooked, with fat ► 32 (Low)
- Cabbage—green, cooked, without fat ► 32 (Low)
- Cabbage—green, raw ► 32 (Low)
- Cabbage—Kim Chee style ► 32 (Low)
- Cabbage—red, cooked, Not Specified as to with fat ► 32 (Low)
- Cabbage—red, cooked, with fat ► 32 (Low)
- Cabbage—red, cooked, without fat ► 32 (Low)
- Cabbage—red, pickled ► 32 (Low)
- Cabbage—red, raw ► 32 (Low)
- Cactus—cooked, Not Specified as to with fat ► 7 (Low)
- Cactus—cooked, with fat ► 7 (Low)
- Cactus—cooked, without fat ► 7 (Low)
- Cactus—raw ► 7 (Low)
- Carrots—canned, low sodium, without fat ► 47 (Low)
- Carrots—cooked, from canned, without fat ► 47 (Low)
- Carrots—cooked, from fresh, without fat ► 47 (Low)

- Carrots—cooked, from frozen, without fat ☛ 47 (Low)
- Carrots—cooked, Not Specified as to form, without fat ☛ 47 (Low)
- Carrots—raw ☛ 16 (Low)
- Cassava—cooked, Not Specified as to with fat ☛ 46 (Low)
- Cassava—cooked, without fat ☛ 46 (Low)
- Cauliflower—cooked, from fresh, without fat ☛ 32 (Low)
- Cauliflower—cooked, from frozen, without fat ☛ 32 (Low)
- Cauliflower—cooked, Not Specified as to form, without fat ☛ 32 (Low)
- Cauliflower—pickled ☛ 32 (Low)
- Cauliflower—raw ☛ 32 (Low)
- Celery juice ☛ 32 (Low)
- Celery—cooked, Not Specified as to with fat ☛ 32 (Low)
- Celery—cooked, with fat ☛ 32 (Low)
- Celery—cooked, without fat ☛ 32 (Low)
- Celery—raw ☛ 32 (Low)
- Chard, cooked, without fat ☛ 32 (Low)
- Chives—raw ☛ 32 (Low)
- Christophine—cooked, without fat ☛ 32 (Low)
- Cilantro—raw ☛ 32 (Low)
- Cocktail sauce ☛ 38 (Low)
- Coleslaw, with dressing ☛ 44 (Low)
- Collards—cooked, from canned, without fat ☛ 32 (Low)
- Collards—cooked, from fresh, without fat ☛ 32 (Low)

THE ESSENTIAL FOODS LISTS FOR THE GLYCEMIC INDEX DIET

- Collards, cooked, from frozen, without fat ☞ 32 (Low)
- Corn relish ☞ 54 (Low)
- Corn—with Pepper— cooked, without fat ☞ 54 (Low)
- Cucumber salad—made with Cucumber—oil, and vinegar ☞ 32 (Low)
- Cucumber salad—with creamy dressing ☞ 32 (Low)
- Cucumber—cooked, Not Specified as to with fat ☞ 32 (Low)
- Cucumber—cooked, with fat ☞ 32 (Low)
- Cucumber—cooked, without fat ☞ 32 (Low)
- Cucumber—pickles, dill ☞ 32 (Low)
- Cucumber—pickles, dill, reduced salt ☞ 32 (Low)
- Cucumber—pickles, fresh ☞ 32 (Low)
- Cucumber—pickles, relish ☞ 32 (Low)
- Cucumber—raw ☞ 32 (Low)
- Cucumber,pickles, sour ☞ 32 (Low)
- Cucumber,pickles, sweet ☞ 32 (Low)
- Dandelion greens—cooked, without fat ☞ 32 (Low)
- Dandelion greens—raw ☞ 32 (Low)
- Dasheen—boiled ☞ 32 (Low)
- Dumpling—potato- or cheese-filled ☞ 52 (Low)
- Eggplant—cooked, Not Specified as to with fat ☞ 32 (Low)
- Eggplant—cooked, tomato sauce, without fat ☞ 35 (Low)
- Eggplant—cooked, with fat ☞ 32 (Low)
- Eggplant—cooked, without fat ☞ 32 (Low)

- Eggplant—pickled ☞ 32 (Low)
- Endive—raw ☞ 32 (Low)
- Escarole—cooked, without fat ☞ 32 (Low)
- Garlic—cooked ☞ 32 (Low)
- Garlic—raw ☞ 32 (Low)
- greens—cooked, from canned, without fat ☞ 32 (Low)
- greens—cooked, from fresh, without fat ☞ 32 (Low)
- Jicama—raw ☞ 32 (Low)
- Kale—cooked, from fresh, without fat ☞ 32 (Low)
- Leek—raw ☞ 32 (Low)
- Lettuce—arugula, raw ☞ 32 (Low)
- Lettuce—Boston, raw ☞ 32 (Low)
- Lettuce—cooked, without fat ☞ 32 (Low)
- Lettuce—raw ☞ 32 (Low)
- Lotus root—cooked, without fat ☞ 32 (Low)
- Mixed salad—greens, raw ☞ 32 (Low)
- Mixed vegetables—corn, lima carrots, beans, peas, and green beans, without fat ☞ 43 (Low)
- Mixed vegetables—from canned, corn, carrots, lima beans, peas, and green beans, cooked, without fat ☞ 43 (Low)
- Mixed vegetables—from corn, carrots, lima beans, peas, and green beans, without fat ☞ 43 (Low)
- Mixed vegetables—from frozen, corn, lima beans, carrots, peas, and green beans, without fat ☞ 43 (Low)
- Mushroom—Oriental, cooked, from dried ☞ 32 (Low)

THE ESSENTIAL FOODS LISTS FOR THE GLYCEMIC INDEX DIET

● Mushrooms—cooked, from canned, Not Specified as to with fat ☛ 32 (Low)

● Mushrooms—cooked, from canned, with fat ☛ 32 (Low)

● Mushrooms—cooked, from canned, without fat ☛ 32 (Low)

● Mushrooms—cooked, from fresh, Not Specified as to with fat ☛ 32 (Low)

● Mushrooms—cooked, from fresh, with fat ☛ 32 (Low)

● Mushrooms—cooked, from fresh, without fat ☛ 32 (Low)

● Mushrooms—cooked, from frozen, Not Specified as to with fat ☛ 32 (Low)

● Mushrooms—cooked, from frozen, with fat ☛ 32 (Low)

● Mushrooms—cooked, Not Specified as to form, Not Specified as to with fat ☛ 32 (Low)

● Mushrooms—cooked, Not Specified as to form, with fat ☛ 32 (Low)

● Mushrooms—cooked, Not Specified as to form, without fat ☛ 32 (Low)

● Mushrooms—pickled ☛ 32 (Low)

● Mushrooms—raw ☛ 32 (Low)

● Mustard greens—cooked, from canned, without fat ☛ 32 (Low)

● Mustard greens—cooked, from fresh, without fat ☛ 32 (Low)

● Mustard greens—cooked, from frozen, without fat ☛ 32 (Low)

● Mustard greens—cooked, Not Specified as to form, without fat ☛ 32 (Low)

● Mustard pickles ☛ 32 (Low)

● Okra—cooked, from canned, with fat ☛ 32 (Low)

- Okra—cooked, from canned, without fat ☞ 32 (Low)
- Okra—cooked, from fresh, Not Specified as to with fat ☞ 32 (Low)
- Okra—cooked, from fresh, with fat ☞ 32 (Low)
- Okra—cooked, from fresh, without fat ☞ 32 (Low)
- Okra—cooked, from frozen, Not Specified as to with fat ☞ 32 (Low)
- Okra—cooked, from frozen, with fat ☞ 32 (Low)
- Okra—cooked, from frozen, without fat ☞ 32 (Low)
- Okra—cooked, Not Specified as to form, Not Specified as to with fat ☞ 32 (Low)
- Okra—cooked, Not Specified as to form, with fat ☞ 32 (Low)
- Okra—cooked, Not Specified as to form, without fat ☞ 32 (Low)
- Okra—pickled ☞ 32 (Low)
- Olives—black ☞ 50 (Low)
- Olives—green ☞ 50 (Low)
- Olives—green, stuffed ☞ 50 (Low)
- Olives—(average value) ☞ 50 (Low)
- Onion, young green, cooked, Not Specified as to form, Not Specified as to with fat ☞ 32 (Low)
- Onions—mature, cooked, from fresh, without fat ☞ 32 (Low)
- Onions—mature, cooked, from frozen, without fat ☞ 32 (Low)
- Onions—mature, cooked, Not Specified as to form, without fat ☞ 32 (Low)
- Onions—mature, raw ☞ 32 (Low)
- Onions—pearl, cooked, from canned ☞ 32 (Low)

THE ESSENTIAL FOODS LISTS FOR THE GLYCEMIC INDEX DIET

- Onions—pearl, cooked, from fresh ► 32 (Low)
- Onions—pearl, cooked, Not Specified as to form ► 32 (Low)
- Onions—young green, cooked, from fresh, without fat ► 32 (Low)
- Onions—young green, cooked, Not Specified as to form, without fat ► 32 (Low)
- Onionscyoung green, raw ► 32 (Low)
- Palm hearts—cooked without fat ► 32 (Low)
- Parsley—cooked without fat ► 32 (Low)
- Parsley—raw ► 32 (Low)
- Peas and Carrots—canned, low sodium, without fat ► 48 (Low)
- Peas and Carrots—cooked, from canned, without fat ► 48 (Low)
- Peas and Carrots—cooked, from fresh, without fat ► 48 (Low)
- Peas and Carrots—cooked, from frozen, without fat ► 48 (Low)
- Peas and Carrots—cooked, Not Specified as to form, without fat ► 48 (Low)
- Peas and corn—cooked, without fat ► 51 (Low)
- Peas and Onions—cooked, without fat ► 40 (Low)
- Peas with Mushrooms—cooked, without fat ► 47 (Low)
- Peas, cowpeas—cooked, from canned, without fat ► 42 (Low)
- Peas, cowpeas—cooked, from fresh, without fat ► 42 (Low)
- Peas, cowpeas—cooked, from frozen, without fat ► 42 (Low)
- Peas, cowpeas—cooked, Not Specified as to form, without fat ► 42 (Low)
- Peas, green—canned, low sodium, without fat ► 48 (Low)

- Peas, green—cooked, from canned, without fat ☛ 48 (Low)
- Peas, green—cooked, from fresh, without fat ☛ 48 (Low)
- Peas, green—cooked, from frozen, without fat ☛ 48 (Low)
- Peas, green—cooked, Not Specified as to form, without fat ☛ 48 (Low)
- Peas, green—raw ☛ 48 (Low)
- Pepper—green, cooked, without fat ☛ 32 (Low)
- Pepper—hot chili, raw ☛ 32 (Low)
- Pepper—hot, cooked, from canned, Not Specified as to with fat ☛ 32 (Low)
- Pepper—hot, cooked, from canned, with fat ☛ 32 (Low)
- Pepper—hot, cooked, from canned, without fat ☛ 32 (Low)
- Pepper—hot, cooked, from fresh, Not Specified as to with fat ☛ 32 (Low)
- Pepper—hot, cooked, from fresh, with fat ☛ 32 (Low)
- Pepper—hot, cooked, from fresh, without fat ☛ 32 (Low)
- Pepper—hot, cooked, from frozen, without fat ☛ 32 (Low)
- Pepper—hot, cooked, Not Specified as to form, Not Specified as to with fat ☛ 32 (Low)
- Pepper—hot, cooked, Not Specified as to form, with fat ☛ 32 (Low)
- Pepper—hot, cooked, Not Specified as to form, without fat ☛ 32 (Low)
- Pepper—hot, pickled ☛ 32 (Low)
- Pepper—pickled ☛ 32 (Low)

- Pepper—poblano, raw 32 (Low)
- Pepper—raw, (average value) 32 (Low)
- Pepper—red, cooked, without fat 32 (Low)
- Pepper—Serrano, raw 32 (Low)
- Pepper—sweet, green, raw 32 (Low)
- Pepper—sweet, red, raw 32 (Low)
- Pigeon peas—cooked, Not Specified as to form, without fat 22 (Low)
- Pimiento 32 (Low)
- Radish—common, raw 32 (Low)
- Radish—Japanese (daikon), cooked, without fat 32 (Low)
- Radish—raw 32 (Low)
- Radishes—pickled, Hawaiian style 32 (Low)
- Recaito (little coriander) 32 (Low)
- Salsa—(average value) 38 (Low)
- Salsa—red, cooked, homemade 38 (Low)
- Salsa—red, cooked, not homemade 38 (Low)
- Salsa—red, uncooked 38 (Low)
- Sauerkraut—canned 32 (Low)
- Sauerkraut—cooked, Not Specified as to with fat 32 (Low)
- Sauerkraut—cooked, with fat 32 (Low)
- Sauerkraut—cooked, without fat 32 (Low)
- Seaweed—dried 32 (Low)
- Seaweed—prepared with soy sauce 32 (Low)

- Seaweed—raw 🡆 32 (Low)
- Snowpea—cooked, from fresh, without fat 🡆 32 (Low)
- Snowpea—cooked, from frozen, without fat 🡆 32 (Low)
- Snowpea—cooked, Not Specified as to form, without fat 🡆 32 (Low)
- Snowpeas raw 🡆 32 (Low)
- Spinach—cooked, from canned, without fat 🡆 32 (Low)
- Spinach—cooked, from fresh, without fat 🡆 32 (Low)
- Spinach—cooked, from frozen, without fat 🡆 32 (Low)
- Spinach—cooked, Not Specified as to form, without fat 🡆 32 (Low)
- Spinach—raw 🡆 32 (Low)
- Sprouts 🡆 32 (Low)
- Squash, spaghetti—cooked, Not Specified as to with fat 🡆 32 (Low)
- Squash, spaghetti—cooked, without fat 🡆 32 (Low)
- Squash, summer—and Onions—cooked, without fat 🡆 32 (Low)
- Squash, summer—cooked, from canned, Not Specified as to with fat 🡆 32 (Low)
- Squash, summer—cooked, from canned, with fat 🡆 32 (Low)
- Squash, summer—cooked, from canned, without fat 🡆 32 (Low)
- Squash, summer—cooked, from fresh, Not Specified as to with fat 🡆 32 (Low)
- Squash, summer—cooked, from fresh, with fat 🡆 32 (Low)
- Squash, summer—cooked, from fresh, without fat 🡆 32 (Low)

THE ESSENTIAL FOODS LISTS FOR THE GLYCEMIC INDEX DIET

- Squash, summer—cooked, from frozen, with fat ➧ 32 (Low)

- Squash, summer—cooked, from frozen, without fat ➧ 32 (Low)

- Squash, summer—cooked, Not Specified as to form, Not Specified as to with fat ➧ 32 (Low)

- Squash, summer—cooked, Not Specified as to form, with fat ➧ 32 (Low)

- Squash, summer—cooked, Not Specified as to form, without fat ➧ 32 (Low)

- Squash, summer—from fresh, creamed ➧ 29 (Low)

- Squash, summer—green, raw ➧ 32 (Low)

- Squash, summer—yellow, raw ➧ 32 (Low)

- Sweetpotato leaves,—cooked, without fat ➧ 32 (Low)

- Sweetpotato with fruit ➧ 53 (Low)

- Tannier—cooked ➧ 32 (Low)

- Taro leaves—cooked, without fat ➧ 32 (Low)

- Taro—baked ➧ 55 (Low)

- Tomato and corn—cooked, without fat ➧ 50 (Low)

- Tomato and Okra—cooked, without fat ➧ 35 (Low)

- Tomato and onion—cooked, Not Specified as to with fat ➧ 35 (Low)

- Tomato and onion, cooked, without fat ➧ 35 (Low)

- Tomato catsup ➧ 38 (Low)

- Tomato chili sauce ➧ 38 (Low)

- Tomato paste ➧ 38 (Low)

- Tomato relish ➧ 32 (Low)

- Tomato—green, pickled ☞ 32 (Low)
- Tomato—green, raw ☞ 38 (Low)
- Tomato—raw ☞ 38 (Low)
- Turnip greens—cooked, from canned, without fat ☞ 32 (Low)
- Turnip greens—cooked, from fresh, without fat ☞ 32 (Low)
- Turnip greens—cooked, from frozen, without fat ☞ 32 (Low)
- Turnip greens—cooked, Not Specified as to form, without fat ☞ 32 (Low)
- Turnip greens—with roots, cooked, from frozen, without fat ☞ 32 (Low)
- Turnip—from fresh, creamed ☞ 40 (Low)
- Vegetable relish ☞ 32 (Low)
- Vegetables—cooked, Not Specified as to with fat, average value ☞ 43 (Low)
- Vegetables—cooked, without fat, average value ☞ 43 (Low)
- Vegetables—pickled ☞ 32 (Low)
- Water chestnut ☞ 32 (Low)
- Watercress—raw ☞ 32 (Low)
- Winter melon—cooked ☞ 32 (Low)
- Yam—cooked ☞ 37 (Low)
- Zucchini—cooked, tomato sauce, without fat ☞ 35 (Low)

HEALTH AND NUTRITION WEBSITES

American Diabetes Association

(www.diabetes.org)

American Heart Association

(www.americanheart.org)

Centers for Disease Control and Prevention

(www.cdc.gov/healthyweight)

Cooking Light

(www.cookinglight.com)

Eating Well

(www.eatingwell.com)

eMedicine Health

(www.emedicinehealth.com)

Fruits and Vegetables Matter

HEALTH AND NUTRITION WEBSITES

(www.fruitsandveggiesmatter.gov)

Health

(www.health.com)

Hormone Foundation

(www.hormone.org)

National Heart, Lung, Blood Institute

(www.nhlbi.nih.gov)

National Institute on Aging

(www.nia.nih.gov)

National Institutes of Health

(http://health.nih.gov)

Nutrition.gov (www.nutrition.gov)

Prevention (www.prevention.com)

ABOUT THE AUTHOR

"Dr. H. Maher" is a joint pen name under which Dr. Y. Naitlho, PharmD, and H. Naitlho, MS/MBA, co-write books.

Dr. Y. Naitlho PharmD has over 25 years of pharmacy practice, applied nutrition research, and writing. He is currently a pharmacist and health and nutrition writer. He is the author of several books in the field of food science and human nutrition, and applied nutrition.

Dr. Y. Naitlho received his Doctor of Pharmacy from Perm State Pharmaceutical Academy. As a pharmacist and nutrition professional, He ensures that book design meets readers' dynamic learning needs and that content meets reliability and integrity standards.

H. Naitlho has over 30 years of engineering practice and science and engineering Research. He is the author of several books in the field of business management and coauthor of numerous books in food science and human nutrition, food engineering, and applied nutrition.

H. Naitlho holds an Engineering degree from the École Supérieure d'Aéronautique et de l'Espace (Sup'Aéro), an Engineering degree from the École de l'Air (Salon de Provence) and has an MBA from Laureate International Universities, a post-graduate degree in Automatics from Paul Sabatier University, and a further post-graduate degree in Mechanics from Aix Marseille University.

H. Naitlho brings the engineering mindset and scientific rigor. He consistently refines ideas, analyzes data, and carries consistency and a great sense of detail to their work.

Printed in Great Britain
by Amazon